Praise for

The SCIENCE *behind* TAPPING

....

"*Dr. Peta Stapleton's* The Science behind Tapping *is a wonderfully thorough review and grounding in Emotional Freedom Techniques (EFT) and other tapping therapies, covering current research, theory, and applications. This book is an important and greatly needed addition to the literature, as well as a handy resource and reference for practitioners, researchers, and consumers.*"

— **Fred P. Gallo, Ph.D., DCEP**, former ACEP president
and author of *Energy Psychology, Energy Tapping for Trauma,*
and *Energy Diagnostic and Treatment Methods*

"*The thousands of people worldwide who have already experienced the incredible trauma release and healing effects of the EFT/tapping therapies know how effective these techniques are. The main barrier to EFT being accepted by mainstream medicine has been the lack of researched-based evidence. In this brilliant book, Dr. Stapleton uses her extensive experience, passion, and drive to bring together this much-needed research information, alongside real-life client experiences.*"

— **Karl Dawson**, EFTMRA director of training, founding EFT
master, author of *Transform Your Beliefs, Transform Your Life*

"The Science behind Tapping *is a much-needed and timely book! It is a treasure trove of all the science and research behind several tapping techniques, written in an easy-to-understand manner. Peta has delivered a vital resource, complete with client stories of the lived experience, that everyone should read.*"

— **Jessica Ortner**, *New York Times* best-selling author of *The
Tapping Solution for Weight Loss and Body Confidence*

"Living in such turbulent times, a book of this caliber is desperately needed as we navigate our way through an abundance of self-care techniques."

— **Kate Helder**, director of Mind Heart Connect

The
SCIENCE
behind
TAPPING

Also by Peta Stapleton, Ph.D.

EFT for Teens

Hay House Titles of Related Interest

YOU CAN HEAL YOUR LIFE, the movie,
starring Louise Hay & Friends
(available as an online streaming video)
www.hayhouse.com/louise-movie

THE SHIFT, the movie,
starring Dr. Wayne W. Dyer
(available as an online streaming video)
www.hayhouse.com/the-shift-movie

. . . .

The EFT Manual, by Dawson Church

The Tapping Solution for Manifesting Your Greatest Self, by Nick Ortner

*The Tapping Solution to Create Lasting Change:
A Guide to Get Unstuck and Find Your Flow,* by Jessica Ortner

*Transform Your Beliefs, Transform Your Life: EFT Tapping
Using Matrix Reimprinting,* by Karl Dawson with Kate Marillat

The

SCIENCE

behind

TAPPING

A PROVEN STRESS MANAGEMENT
TECHNIQUE FOR THE
MIND & BODY

DR. PETA STAPLETON, Ph.D.

HAY HOUSE, INC.
Carlsbad, California • New York City
London • Sydney • New Delhi

Published in the United States by: Hay House, Inc.: www.hayhouse.com®
Published in Australia by: Hay House Australia Pty. Ltd.: www.hayhouse.com.au
Published in the United Kingdom by: Hay House UK, Ltd.: www.hayhouse.co.uk
Published in India by: Hay House Publishers India: www.hayhouse.co.in

Indexer: Jay Kreider • *Cover design:* Howie Severson • *Interior design:* Pamela Homan

Library of Congress has cataloged the earlier edition as follows:

Names: Stapleton, Peta.
Title: The science behind tapping : a proven stress management technique for the mind & body / Peta Stapleton, Ph.D.
Description: 1st edition. | Carlsbad, California : Hay House, Inc., 2019. | Includes bibliographical references and index.
Identifiers: LCCN 2018059648| ISBN 9781401955731 (hardcover : alk. paper) | ISBN 9781401955755 (ebook)
Subjects: LCSH: Emotional Freedom Techniques. | Stress management. | Mind and
body therapies.
Classification: LCC RC489.E45 S728 2019 | DDC 616.89/1--dc23 LC record available at https://lccn.loc.gov/2018059648

Tradepaper ISBN: 978-1-4019-5574-8
Audiobook ISBN: 978-1-4019-6367-5
E-book ISBN: 978-1-4019-5575-5

10 9 8 7 6 5 4 3 2 1
1st edition, April 2019
2nd edition, January 2022

SUSTAINABLE
FORESTRY
INITIATIVE
Certified Chain of Custody
Promoting Sustainable Forestry
www.sfiprogram.org
SFI-01268
SFI label applies to the text stock

Printed in the United States of America

For Megan and Elise:

*Love you
to the moon
and back.*

CONTENTS

....

AUTHOR'S NOTE

Although they are gaining in scientific support, Emotional Freedom Techniques (EFT) and "tapping" are still considered experimental in nature. All information, books, workshops, and trainings are intended to promote awareness of the benefits of learning and applying EFT. However, the general public must take full responsibility for their use of it. The material in this book is for your general knowledge only and is not a substitute for traditional medical attention, counseling, therapy, or advice from a qualified health-care professional.

Neither EFT nor the information here is intended to be used to diagnose, treat, cure, or prevent any disease or disorder. Please note that if you begin tapping and find yourself overwhelmed, distressed, or becoming aware of previously forgotten memories, you may need to seek the professional help of a trained and experienced EFT practitioner.

A lack of results or progress may also mean you need professional assistance. If you have any concern regarding your health or mental state, it is recommended that you seek out advice or treatment from a qualified, licensed health-care professional. Before making any changes to your diet, medication, or health plan, it is recommended that you first consult with a doctor, pharmacist, or other qualified medical or health professional.

All names and identifying details of real clients have been changed to protect their privacy.

FOREWORD

In an age of information, ignorance is a choice. With the advent of technology, we as human beings are freer in so many ways. We no longer need a teacher or a formal education to gain access to information that was once only at the hands of authorities and experts. By the same means, people all over the world are more empowered to proactively research a diagnosis and initiate significant lifestyle changes, and even seek alternative treatments for their health condition—without consulting a doctor and blindly taking a medication—and they are having considerable results. Others are taking the time to delve deep into well-researched understandings about ancient religions, theology, and the nature of reality without a priest, a minister, or a rabbi—and they are having profound mystical experiences that change them for the rest of their lives. EFT (Emotional Freedom Techniques), or tapping, has become one such way people are transforming their beliefs, their emotions, and their lives. Information is literally at our fingertips with the self-applied technique of tapping, and it affords us the ability to make new, different, and better choices.

When you learn information, the understanding of new knowledge creates a greater sense of awareness about yourself as well as the world around you. It lifts you above the mundane, routine way you see the world. A new awareness about some "thing" creates a new level of consciousness, and when there is a change in consciousness, there is a change in energy. As a result, you become empowered and more awakened by knowledge because knowledge has always been powerful. Thus, when you learn knowledge about yourself, you are empowering yourself. In a sense, you are taking your power back by no longer believing you are a helpless victim who believes you have no power to change; or you cease being someone who keeps unconsciously giving your power away to (or relying on) someone or something to do it for you. We are living in a new era of consciousness.

From a neuroscientific standpoint, learning is making new synaptic connections. Every time you learn something new, your brain assembles thousands of new circuits which are reflected as patterns in your gray matter. In fact, the latest brain science research demonstrates that when you focus your attention for one hour on one concept or idea, the number of connections in your brain literally doubles. These new footprints of consciousness are the physical evidence that you learned by interacting with your environment.

However, the same research shows that if you don't repeatedly think about what you've learned, or you never take the time to review the new information over and over again, those circuits will prune apart within hours or days. If learning is making new synaptic connections, then remembering is maintaining or sustaining those new connections. Tapping works in a similar way when change has occurred. Once the tapping technique has resolved your concern, then it rarely needs to be done again on the same issue. The neural pathways change, and that old behavior, thought, or feeling is a distant memory.

Knowledge changes you. With just a little concentration and repetition, intellectual information becomes embossed in your biology. Learning (and remembering) causes you to no longer see things the way *they are,* but the way *you are.* A different lens of how you perceive the world is inserted into your brain and as a consequence, you see new possibilities that you were unaware of before your interaction with knowledge. That's because your brain only sees equal to how it is wired. And that means you can only see what you know.

In the research I've conducted with literally thousands and thousands of people all over the world, I now know that once a person understands an idea, a concept, or new information—and they can turn to the person next to them and explain that information—they are firing and wiring certain circuits in their brain. These circuits add new stitches into the three-dimensional tapestry of their brain's neural architecture, allowing them to successfully wire the circuits necessary to initiate that new knowledge into a new experience. In other words, once you can remember and discuss the new model of understanding, you are beginning to install the neurological hardware in preparation for an experience.

The more you know what you're doing and why, the *how* gets easier. That's why this is a time in history when it's not enough to simply *know*—it's a time to *know how*. Your next job is to initiate that knowledge by applying, personalizing, or demonstrating what you philosophically and theoretically learned. This means you're going to have to make new and different choices—and get your body involved. And when you can align your behaviors with your intentions, you are going to have a new experience.

Once you embrace a new experience, the new event will add to (and further enhance) the intellectual circuitry in your brain. It's a fact that experience enriches the synaptic connections. The moment those circuits further organize into new networks, the brain makes a chemical. That chemical is called a feeling or an emotion. That means the instant you feel freedom, wholeness, or joy from that novel event, now you're teaching your body chemically to understand what your mind has intellectually understood. Now new information is making its way to your body—not just your mind—and it's changing your state of being. This is often the reason people say they feel calm, peaceful and even deliriously happy after they have used tapping—the brain changes, and long-term follow-up trials are showing it *stays* changed.

It's fair to say then that knowledge is for the mind and experience is for the body. Now you are beginning to *embody the truth* of that philosophy. In doing so, you're rewriting your biological program and signaling new genes in new ways. That's because new information is coming from the environment. As we know from epigenetics, if the environment signals new genes, and the end-product of an experience in the environment is an emotion, you are literally signaling the new genes in new ways. Now you're beginning to chemically instruct your body to understand what your mind has theoretically understood. And since all genes make proteins, and proteins are responsible for the structure and function of your body (the expression of proteins is the expression of life), you are literally changing your genetic destiny. This suggests that it's quite possible your body can be healed in a moment.

If you can create an experience once, you should be able to do it again. When you can reproduce any experience over and over again, eventually you will neuro-chemically condition your mind and body to begin to work as one. When you've done something so many times that the body knows how to do it as well as the mind, it becomes automatic, natural, and effortless—simply said, now it has become a skill or a habit. Once you've achieved that level, you no longer have to consciously think about doing it. That's when the skill or habit becomes the subconscious state of being. Now it's innate and you're beginning to *master that philosophy*. You have become that knowledge.

This is how common people around the world are waking up and beginning to do—what has been considered for thousands of years—the uncommon. In doing so they are transitioning from philosopher to initiate to master; from knowledge to experience to wisdom; from mind to body to soul; from thinking to doing to being; and from learning with their head, practicing it by hand, and knowing it by heart. The beauty of it is, we all have the biological and neurological machinery to do this.

The side effect of your repeated efforts will not only change who you are, but it should create even more possibilities in your life that are a reflection your efforts. Why else would you do it? What do I mean when I say possibilities? I'm talking about healing from diseases and imbalances of both the body as well as the mind, creating a better life by no longer making the same unconscious choices that were programmed from past traumas. The result may be a new job, a new relationship, a new opportunity, and new adventures in life; as well as a complete recovery of long-term addictions, subconscious cravings, and hardwired self-destructive habits.

And that's what this powerful book is all about. *The Science behind Tapping* is your personal guide to prove to yourself how powerful you truly are when you apply what you are about to learn. It was written for you to not just intellectually understand the content but to consistently use the practices and apply them to your life so that you reap the rewards of your efforts—not only for you, but for your family and friends as well.

It's no short order to find the funding to do any research—especially research that does not entail creating a new drug for profit. It's equally challenging to create a solid working hypothesis and perform the proper type of gold standard research, using functional brain technology and other objective measurements to test efficacy. It takes hours of investigation, examination, and preparation to create a scientific model of understanding that proves that our mind and body work as one. And it takes a Herculean effort to organize, disseminate, and find meaning in the results of a broad range of scientific findings—never mind write a book about it. Yet, my dear friend and colleague Peta Stapleton has taken this task on in this fantastically well-written book.

I first met Peta at a research conference that she was holding on the Gold Coast of Australia in 2017. I was prepped by my colleagues that she was an excellent empirical scientist. I was told that she had strict standards on investigative research. And of course, I was presenting my research at her conference and I was a bit uncertain about what to expect. I thought, *Should I prepare for the worst? If I am challenged on my research, how should I defend it?* Science can be a bitter game of egos.

When I met Peta, she was nothing like my mind had conjured up. We had an instant connection. She is intelligent, charismatic, heart-centered, loving, joyful, kind, cooperative, friendly, and she communicates very well. Peta loves knowledge and she is certainly not afraid to investigate and then stand up for information that flies in the face of convention—and she's smart enough to prove it correct—or incorrect. As a scientist, she has been a pioneer in the Energy Psychology genre before it became mainstream.

Peta is resource of knowledge and experience—and as you just learned, that leads to wisdom. She is the leading expert in the art, science, and philosophy of EFT. She has spent many years asking the right questions, then finding the best answers. She knows her material very well.

Peta and I share the same passion—to understand and to know more about who we really are and what is possible for human beings, especially during these modern times. Her work and research has directly and indirectly changed thousands of lives.

I loved reading this book because it provided answers to some of my own personal questions about the relationship between the mind and the body. I learned new concepts and it helped me see the world differently. I was changed from my time reading it. In fact, I found myself tapping on all kinds of things the entire time I was studying it. I was deeply engaged in the book on a 10-hour flight from London to Los Angeles, I think I tapped on at least 50 different items and found myself mystified by how different I felt. I thought to myself: *It works! I feel different.* I smiled because I was literally embodying knowledge as truth.

It is my hope that, not only will this masterpiece of knowledge and experience change you as well as help you to see the world differently, but it will also inspire you to apply the principles so that you embody the truth of what is possible for you in your life.

You are about to learn from someone who has gone from philosopher to initiate to master.

Peta Stapleton is the master of her craft.

Dr. Joe Dispenza, *New York Times* best-selling author of
You Are the Placebo: Making Your Mind Matter

INTRODUCTION

....

"Tapping" was introduced as a key element of a self-help approach in the 1970s. Since then, the popularity of this easy-to-apply, yet incredibly effective tool for stress regulation and personal transformation has grown and grown. Pitched originally as a psychotherapy technique to address emotional problems, its most widely used and best-researched format is known as the Emotional Freedom Techniques, or simply EFT.

With roots in Eastern philosophies, particularly acupuncture, our understanding of *how* EFT works has been rapidly progressing. While initial explanations focused on the body's meridian system, we now understand that EFT has profound effects on the nervous system, the production of stress hormones (particularly cortisol), DNA regulation, and brain activation.

Put simply, we have come a long way.

This book is designed to unpack all the research, which began in the 1990s, and present it in an easy-to-read manner. It also clearly outlines what happens when you use EFT. EFT Universe, one of several EFT websites worldwide, is home to over 5,000 individual case studies, but we now have much more than just anecdotal reports showcasing EFT's effectiveness. Further evidence of that effectiveness can now be found in more than 100 outcome studies; clinical reports; review articles; randomized clinical trials; head-to-head comparisons with gold standard therapies; and the ultimate in research, meta-analyses. A comprehensive review of the research on tapping concluded that independent investigations in more than a dozen countries have consistently demonstrated strong positive outcomes after relatively few treatment sessions. Conditions responding well included phobias, anxiety, depression, and post-traumatic stress disorder (PTSD).

Because one of the core techniques of EFT is to stimulate selected points on the face and upper body by tapping on them, EFT is commonly also called "tapping." For this reason, you will find that many researchers, including myself, use the phrases *EFT* and *tapping* interchangeably. In fact, the word *tapping* has become an easy-to-comprehend explanation of EFT, popularized by Nick Ortner and Jessica Ortner of The Tapping Solution (www .thetappingsolution.com).

But first things first: How did I, a mainstream clinical and health psychologist, come to use this tool in the 1990s? Why did I find myself doing research on such a new and very different field?

MY STORY

As a natural listener, I felt called to the field of psychology to help others. After graduating with a traditional psychology degree, I felt like I was on top of the world. I started to specialize in eating disorders such as anorexia and bulimia nervosa. I was conducting free weekly support groups and individual sessions, and started teaching at a local university. But something was missing.

No matter what I used from my clinical training, my clients weren't improving fast enough for their (or my) satisfaction. I was starting to feel like a failure. Granted I was still young and green as a therapist, but I was disillusioned and beginning to panic that these sufferers were being left out in the cold by the field because "nothing worked" for them. It was at this stage that a colleague reached out. He had been surfing the "Net" and had come across something that he thought would help.

When he pitched it to me, he said, "I've found a technique that I think might work, but it's a little bit weird." Now *that* didn't land very well. I was a serious psychologist and not into weird things! But desperation leads to desperate measures, so I invited him to come along to one of the eating-disorder support groups. During that particular session, one of the young participants started to have a panic attack. My colleague gestured that he would take her to another room to help her calm while I kept teaching. Less than 15 minutes later, they were both back. The young woman had gone from panicked and hyperventilating to calm and composed. My eyebrows started touching the ceiling.

After the group ended and everyone had left, I was eager to find out what he did. He said, "I did that weird tapping thing I told you about." Of course I needed to know more!

As the year went on, I began learning about EFT. As one tends to do when excited about a new discovery, I started using it with friends and family and of course on myself. I attended a practical training and used the technique on my craving for chocolate. Now, 20 years later, I still have no desire for chocolate. I used to eat it daily for an afternoon energy boost, so this was no mean feat. I can still eat chocolate (tapping doesn't remove free will), but I barely enjoy it and never want more than one bite.

When my job description changed at my university around the early 2000s, I found myself in a position where I had to conduct research. I was still working in the field of eating disorders, and by this time had been successfully using EFT with clients for many years. I was not telling many people about the technique; however, my clients were recovering! So I broached the idea of researching EFT for eating issues with my very conservative supervisor at the time, a medical practitioner. He said, "Sounds interesting, but I don't think anyone will come to the trial."

I decided to move forward anyway. We had settled on using it for food cravings in overweight adults, since the obesity epidemic in Australia at that time was alarming. (We also thought that more people would attend in this category rather than for anorexia or bulimia nervosa. In clinical trials, sample size is very important for establishing the significance of the findings.) We received a small grant from the Association for Comprehensive Energy Psychology in the United States—a huge act of faith as their committee knew nothing about me or my team and probably wondered who we were! I also reached out to a national current-affairs television program and was filmed for a story on the trial. We were offering a free four-week, eight-hour program to learn EFT for food cravings, and I demonstrated the technique on air with the interviewer and his chocolate muffin.

Well, the response was wild. We received over 4,500 calls and e-mails from around the country with people wanting to join the trial. (My manager couldn't believe it!) I knew we might be at the start of something big.

The rest is history. We went on to conduct that trial with 120 adults. Over the next decade, we extended our research by comparing EFT with established gold standard therapies and adapted it for youth and other populations and conditions. About three years after the first current-affairs program, I called that reporter and offered him the story of the follow-up from the trial. Everything we had measured had changed with EFT, and a year later the improvements remained! (See Chapter 7 for our results.)

He said to me, "I don't know what you did that day three years ago, but I still can't eat a chocolate muffin." I had to laugh.

So I have continued to test this interesting and fairly new technique in research trials. We have now also examined EFT for chronic pain, major depression, fear of failure in high-achieving students, and cigarette smoking, and the efficacy of delivering EFT services online. To be clear, I know many traditional therapies work. I am an associate professor at a university and program director in the master of clinical psychology program; and in my classes, I teach every mainstream, evidence-based therapy you read about. But, and there is a *but*, even approaches that are supported by research do not have the "one size fits all" quality enjoyed by EFT.

Of course a claim like that needs to be validated by research. Anecdotal evidence can be powerful if you trust your neighbor who suggests that you try a particular approach, but our patients need to know whether a therapy they are considering has been empirically tested and its effectiveness established. The questions about EFT that are most interesting to me as a psychologist are whether EFT works, and whether it works for a wide range of individuals and conditions, as I suspect. We are also curious whether the encouraging clinical outcomes we are seeing might be due to factors other than the tapping.

I have now become Australia's main EFT researcher, and I continue to be amazed by how quickly our participants' lives improve. I believe we will teach this clinical tool as a mainstream technique at university level in the not-so-far-off future, and I truly look forward to that day.

So this brings us to this question: Where does EFT sit in relation to traditional therapies, and why might the world be about to embrace it?

A FOURTH WAVE!

Individual psychotherapy is considered to have developed in three great waves. In the field's early days, we had psychoanalysis. You are perhaps familiar with the pioneering giants of this movement, such as Sigmund Freud and Carl Jung. They emphasized unconscious conflicts, early experiences, and the "transference" of feelings from the patient's childhood onto the therapist. Researchers and proponents of behavior modification followed. Early leaders, such as Edward Thorndike, Joseph Wolpe, and B. F. Skinner, drew upon learning theory to formulate strategies for changing unwanted behaviors. Using positive and negative reinforcers (called contingencies), they were able to measurably increase desirable behaviors and extinguish self-defeating behavioral patterns in their clients.

Emerging from psychoanalysis and behavioral therapies came two movements that each considered itself a "third wave." Humanistic or experiential psychotherapy challenged core tenets of psychoanalysis and behaviorism, such as the idea that every event is determined by an unbroken chain of prior occurrences. It instead stressed the inherent goodness of each individual and the possibility of reaching toward this potential by supporting qualities such as free will, creativity, self-esteem, love, and autonomy.

While the humanistic movement is no longer a major force within the field, it has left its mark on most contemporary psychotherapeutic approaches.

Meanwhile, cognitive therapy or cognitive behavioral therapy (since it builds on behavior therapy) emerged as another "third wave," and it has by now become the dominant force in psychotherapy. Cognitive therapy targets a client's thoughts and interpretations of situations, as these can result in negative emotional states. Pioneers in this area include Aaron Beck and Judith Beck, Albert Ellis, and David Burns. A recent development within cognitive therapy has been a shift of emphasis from the symptoms caused by faulty cognitive appraisals (the way you think) to deeper changes in thought processes through witnessing, accepting, and being with the ongoing flow of inner experience. These newer approaches include mindfulness, acceptance and commitment therapy, dialectical behavior therapy, and blends such as mindfulness-integrated cognitive behavioral therapy.

Historically, psychotherapy has been a very long process. But the need for briefer treatments is being pushed for obvious economic reasons so that the wide range of people who could benefit from psychotherapy can have a chance of receiving it. Insurance plans and subsidized treatment such as Medicare often have limitations on the number of sessions that can be accessed in any one calendar year. This has resulted in an upsurge of research on briefer approaches, which are generally regarded as therapies that require more than 2 but fewer than 10 sessions.

Many of the most successful brief treatment models utilize somatic interventions, including movement, sensory stimulation and integration, or the activation of areas on the skin, such as acupoints (areas important in acupuncture), that set into motion desired neurological processes. The emergence of brief psychotherapies that include a somatic component are now being considered psychotherapy's fourth wave. For instance, Eye Movement Desensitization and Reprocessing (EMDR) is recognized as an empirically validated treatment for trauma, anxiety, and depression.[1] I consider EFT to be the most promising of the fourth-wave psychotherapies I have investigated.

HOW THIS BOOK IS ORGANIZED

The Science behind Tapping is designed for a wide range of readers. Those who are interested in EFT for self-help and are curious to learn what is actually known about the method will find an abundance of current, authoritative information. Clinicians and researchers who want to see the evidence for the method's efficacy and how research findings can inform its practice will find that the information and claims presented are backed by relevant, informative studies.

Many case studies are included in each chapter so you can hear from the clients themselves. The lived experience of sufferers is not to be underestimated with any therapeutic approach and often informs us on how to improve.

Before I talk about how to get the most out of this book, here is an overview of each chapter and what will be covered.

Chapter 1 explores what EFT actually is and why we call it tapping. We discuss EFT in terms of it being a stress-reduction tool or self-help technique that calms your mind. (When I am talking in the media, I often say EFT is similar to "psychological acupuncture.") This chapter also contains a beginner's guide to EFT and walks you through how to use it. Handouts to match this chapter are available on my website: www.petastapleton.com.

Chapter 2 considers why you would consider using EFT. It briefly discusses the history of where the technique came from, the different versions that exist, and why we actually tend to only investigate Clinical EFT in the trials we run.

Chapter 3 opens with the mounting research behind EFT across a range of areas. Please note that not every EFT study that has ever been conducted is included in this book. Mostly I present the most credible research that has had the largest impact in the field, with the aim of giving you the best picture of the outcomes.

This chapter considers the single case studies that started the process and how these grew into clinical trials, and now meta-analyses (this means so many trials have been conducted in one area that we can develop a single conclusion that has the greater statistical power). While psychological trials typically use measurements of self-report, in which a participant subjectively indicates their mood state and so on through a questionnaire, the studies of tapping have now expanded to measure physiological changes, such as cortisol levels and DNA expression. We also have the first neural brain scans of EFT treatment, and more of these studies are underway.

Chapter 4 focuses on EFT and PTSD. This is an exciting chapter because, to date, this area has probably had the most EFT research conducted. It is suggested 8 out of every 100 people will have PTSD at some point in their lives; this rate is higher in military personnel.[2] I overview the symptoms and causes of PTSD and the effects it has on the brain at various ages. Because some research has focused on the physiological changes after tapping with PTSD, I explore these studies as well as the psychological benefits that have been reported. We now know that genes in sufferers of PTSD can be transformed through EFT, and these changes last over time. This chapter also offers case examples of participants who have benefitted from tapping.

Chapter 5 explores EFT, stress, and anxiety. In the United States, anxiety affects about 18 percent of the population, yet only about a third of these individuals receive any treatment.[3] This is despite the fact that it is considered a highly treatable condition. The World Health Organization has said that between 1990 and 2013, the number of people suffering from depression and/or anxiety increased by nearly 50 percent. In addition, mental disorders are accounting for 30 percent of the global nonfatal disease burden.[4] With this in mind, this chapter outlines the research investigating the effect of EFT on stress and anxiety. Real case studies, notes from practitioners, and research on specific areas are presented.

Chapter 6 then delves into using EFT for depression. This condition is considered the leading cause of ill health and disability worldwide, with more than 300 million people living with this debilitating condition, and an increase of more than 18 percent between 2005 and 2015.[5] It is vital we have a wider range of evidence-based solutions. This chapter not only discusses the research trials and outcomes, but also shows how using EFT for other conditions (e.g., food cravings) also reduces depressive symptoms. Participant stories and practical tips are offered throughout.

Chapter 7 summarizes how tapping can be used for food cravings and weight issues. We have over a decade of clinical trials that clearly show the effectiveness of tapping for reducing food cravings in overweight and obese adults, leading to weight loss over time. These studies have a minimum of one-year follow-up, which means it is easier to see the effectiveness lasting over time. This is the one area where we have neural brain scans that show the difference in the brain's activity before and after an EFT treatment program, and the results are extraordinarily exciting. (Even the radiologist on the team couldn't quite believe it!) Because this is my particular area of research, there are many participant stories and concrete recommendations for using with clients or yourself.

Chapter 8 covers how to use tapping with children and adolescents and the outcomes of the investigations to date. This is a growing area of research focus and extends into school and academic issues, therefore this chapter explores common student issues (e.g., perfectionism, test anxiety) as well as learning disabilities. I present how tapping can be effectively used in a classroom and the home environment, and include practitioner and participant stories. The next generation may truly benefit from this stress-reduction tool, and using it as a daily option in school situations is proving to be a worthy addition to any curriculum. The clinical trials are demonstrating solid outcomes for children and teens, and this will be an exciting area to watch in the future.

Chapter 9 examines other conditions that have been the focus of research and testing, including phobias, obsessive-compulsive disorder, chronic pain and fibromyalgia, physical and emotional issues, addiction, and various medical conditions such as breast cancer and brain injury. Several practitioners share practical sessions throughout this chapter to offer insight into how people's lives are transformed with tapping.

Chapter 10 highlights other tapping techniques that have featured in research trials. These include the forerunner to EFT, Thought Field Therapy; a hybrid called Matrix Reimprinting; and other trauma tapping techniques. These approaches still use the key ingredients in EFT, but may have additional aspects. A range of topics is included in this chapter, from PTSD to public speaking.

Chapter 11 wraps things up with a discussion of common obstacles to your success with EFT. While the research clearly offers the evidence for the effectiveness of tapping, in a noisy online world, there may still be accounts of why EFT doesn't or didn't work for someone. This chapter explores why this happens and what to do if tapping appears not to be working. It also offers a summary of common rookie mistakes. The last section here describes how to discuss EFT in a scientific, evidence-based way to newcomers or professional colleagues, and even the media. After 20 years in the field, I have learned what "lands" and what doesn't, and how to build a bridge to existing knowledge.

The book ends with how you can learn more about EFT and where to go to follow future research. All references are offered in full at the end and details of research giants to follow and important resources are included.

HOW TO GET THE MOST OUT OF THIS BOOK

If you are new to EFT and just starting out, I would highly recommend reading from beginning to end. It will give you a solid account of this technique and how to use it, and then the evidence from the trials.

If you are an existing practitioner or researcher and very familiar with the practical application of tapping, then you may be interested in choosing to read from Chapter 3 onward. This will contribute to your knowledge of the empirically validated trials and highlight the effectiveness of EFT to similar and existing gold standard psychological approaches.

If you have a particular interest in any single topic, you can go straight to that chapter.

Let's begin.

WHAT IS EFT?

While EFT can address a range of complex emotional challenges, the basic protocol is quite straightforward and surprisingly easy to learn. It instructs you on only two activities: *what you say or think* and *where you tap*. It is a powerful way to come to terms with unresolved childhood issues, change unwanted responses to various emotional triggers, transform beliefs that do not serve you, and reprogram yourself for greater happiness and success.

What you say or think during an EFT session involves an ever-shifting focus on (1) your initial concern, (2) its roots in your history, (3) the feelings and sensations it creates in your body, and (4) self-suggestions or affirmations about what you want to change.

Where you tap is based on the ancient system of acupuncture. Certain acupoints (areas important in acupuncture) have been shown to have a powerful impact on the way the brain responds to stress and the way it processes information.

Note that the technique outlined in this chapter represents Clinical EFT. This is the version mostly tested in research trials. (Researchers worldwide tend to use only Clinical EFT in their trials, because it is only in establishing evidence for a defined protocol that we can then extend it to briefer or adapted versions.)

HOW TO TAP

Acupoints on the face and upper body are stimulated in EFT by tapping on them with two fingers; usually the index and middle fingers. The amount of force used while tapping should be firm yet always comfortable. You may feel a resonance spreading out across the adjacent area of your body from the point you are tapping, but even if you don't feel it, it is still occurring. Some instructions suggest that you should tap on each spot about seven times before moving on to the next, but you don't need to count since you will tap for as long as it takes to say the statement you formulate at each point.

Tapping can be used to change distressing or negative feelings and self-limiting thoughts or behaviors as well as to instill more positive emotional states, beliefs, or goals. Typically, you clear any distressing or negative aspects with tapping before using it to open up more positive possibilities in that area.

THE STEPS

Here are the five basic steps of EFT:

1. First recognize what you wish to change and rate your distress/discomfort about this area of your life on a scale of 0 to 10 (10: extreme distress; 0: no distress). This is called the "subjective units of distress" (SUD) rating. It is an internal assessment about the intensity of your feelings around the problem, and it is fine if it just feels like a guess. Your intuition will guide you. The aim is to tap until you feel calmer about the issue, and usually the number will go down to 0 or 1. You can also stop with a higher SUD rating if the shift you have achieved feels like enough for that particular EFT session.

2. Next you capture the problem in a *setup statement* (see the next section), which you state while tapping on

the side-of-the-*hand point* (see Figure 1A). While you can state it in your mind, you may be more likely to drift in your thoughts. Plus saying it out loud engages you more fully with the statement.

3. Next tap through all eight EFT points on the face and upper body (see Figure 1B) while saying a short *reminder phrase* to keep your mind engaged. This is usually a word or brief phrase that describes your feeling in relation to the setup statement. Tapping on the eight points is called a *round* in EFT.

4. Take a breath and re-rate your distress between 0 and 10 on the SUD scale. Remember this can be a subjective, intuitive guess. It is better to use the first number that comes into your mind than to ponder it too long.

5. Keep tapping through additional rounds (using the face and upper body points) until the SUD rating is quite low, a 1 or 0.

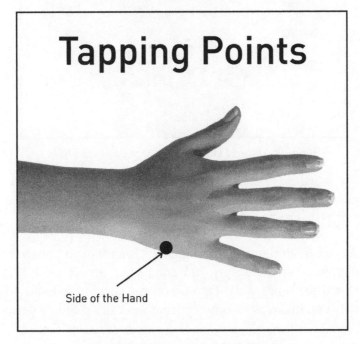

Figure 1A: Tapping point on side of hand

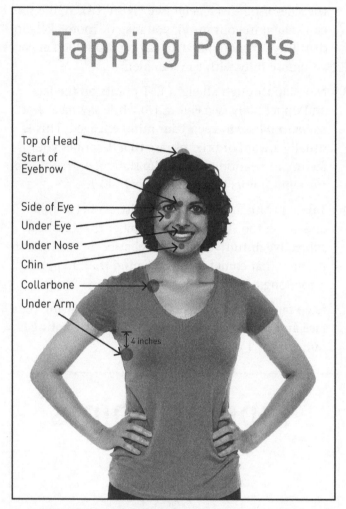

Figure 1B: The eight EFT points on the face and upper body

THE SETUP STATEMENT

A typical setup statement might be: "Even though I [insert your feeling/issue here], I deeply and completely accept myself." You say this three times while tapping on the side-of-the-hand point. There is a saying in psychotherapy that you can't change a personal quality unless you first accept it, and this pairing of your problem with an acceptance statement helps build that self-acceptance. Because you are focusing on your feeling, the setup statement keeps you in the present moment.

While you can change the ending of the setup statement, it should accomplish two things:

- State the actual problem or feeling.

- Express acceptance that this is how you currently feel—*right now* (even though you are aiming to change the feeling or the situation that evokes the feeling).

With that in mind, you could say any of the following at the end of the setup statement:

- Even though I . . . , I accept I have this problem.

- Even though I . . . , I am still a good person.

- Even though I . . . , I am taking charge right now.

- Even though I . . . , I want to change this.

- Even though I . . . , I completely and sincerely accept myself.

- Even though I . . . , I completely love/like and accept myself.

- Even though I . . . , I deeply and completely love and accept myself anyway.

- Even though I . . . , I deeply and completely forgive myself.

- Even though I . . . , I deeply and completely love and accept my feelings.

- Even though I . . . , I choose to love and accept myself.

- Even though I . . . , I choose to be open to this process.

- Even though I . . . , I am okay and open to the process.

- Even though I . . . , right here right now, I am safe.

In brief, the opening part of the setup statement includes a short description of the problem or your feelings about it. Then, in the second part, you are giving yourself an affirmation or self-suggestion that you recognize and accept *what is*. This focus on "what is" is a feature of mindfulness, which has proven to be a highly effective practice when introduced into the therapy setting. Meanwhile, tapping on the acupoints helps calm the brain, making it even easier to stay in the present moment.

The emphasis on accepting the problem and your feelings about it may seem counterintuitive. You might wonder, *Why not just focus on the desired changes?* However, self-help and therapeutic approaches that begin by "attacking" the problem or one's patterns of thought and emotion tend to bring up inner resistance that undermines the approach.

Using "I Choose" Statements

Dr. Patricia Carrington pioneered the "I choose" statements to help make the beneficial changes from EFT to become permanent and generalize to many aspects of your life.[1] Try this by adding "I choose" to the end of the setup statement. Here are examples of how this is included:

- "Even though I feel my mother never loved me, I choose to love myself anyway."

- "Even though I feel deprived when I don't have chocolate, I choose to be fit and healthy."

- "Even though I'm nervous about giving that talk on Tuesday, I choose to be calm and confident."

So Why Do We State the Negative?

This is a common question, as many therapies seek to reframe a person's issue, or simply learn to accept it. Tapping doesn't affirm or implant a problem; however, on the surface it may look like that. The process does have someone state the *truth* of what is happening for him or her and acknowledge it. We are actually engaging the amygdala (stress center) and the limbic system (emotions) in the brain and body with this technique.

It is as though we are engaging these negative feelings or sensations just long enough to feel them, then we hit the delete button through the tapping.

It is the tapping process that calms the physiological response from the body. Once this is released, cognitive shifts (or reframes) may surface naturally.

If we tap with a positive affirmation first (attempting to take our mind off our problem), it may only result in a minor shift. It is like spraying air freshener when the garbage is still there. We need to tap on the real problem and reduce the intensity before tapping on anything positive—there is more on how to tap on the positive later in this chapter.

The key in EFT is to actually do the tapping when you acknowledge your problem and state it out loud. It is the somatic aspect that changes the response, not just stating your problem. There have been several comparison studies of the active ingredient of EFT done, often by researchers who do not use the technique at all, and these are discussed in Chapter 3. Basically we now know that the tapping aspect is a key active ingredient in the process working—and just stating your problem with an acceptance element may not result in it changing.

REMINDER PHRASE

The short reminder phrase you say as you tap on each acu-point captures the main feeling or negative state you want to change (e.g., "angry" or "sad").

Suppose you will be giving a talk next week, and you are nervous about it. To apply EFT, you would start with a setup statement such as this:

"Even though I'm feeling anxious and nervous about the talk I have to give, I accept this is how I feel right now."

Your reminder phrase could be "nervous" or "anxious." This is the feeling you would initially rate on its intensity from 0 to 10, and then rate again after each round of tapping. This gives you instant feedback about what is happening as a result of that tapping round.

You will usually find that the SUD rating has gone down, but occasionally it will have increased. This generally means you have tuned in to the problem more deeply rather than that tapping hasn't worked. When this occurs, the true SUD was always the higher number, and you continue from there.

Ideally you should keep tapping as long as your SUD rating is still more than 1. You can adjust the reminder phrase if you think of a better description as you tap. For instance, you might start by using "angry" as your main feeling, but after a few rounds of tapping, you may realize the feeling is now disappointment. So "disappointed" would become your reminder phrase.

SAMPLE SESSION OF TAPPING

Here is how I might proceed through a session of tapping if I had a headache.

First, I recognize my headache and rate the throbbing pain as a 9 out of 10 on the SUD scale.

I then tap on the side of my hand with two fingers of the other hand (see Figure 1A) while saying, "Even though I have this headache in both temples and feel sick, I accept that I have this headache." I do this three times while tapping on the side-of-the-hand point.

Then I would start tapping through the eight points (see Figure 1B) and say, "This headache" or "I feel sick." I could also use descriptive words, such as "throbbing pain."

I would repeat the rounds of tapping until I felt a shift or difference, usually indicated by a low SUD number. Then the session would be complete.

POSITIVE TAPPING

Although most people tap only when they discover a negative feeling they would like to reduce or change, you can use tapping for positive statements. Do this only *after* you have reduced any negative feelings associated with a memory, thought, or feeling. You can then do rounds of positive tapping to introduce any new feeling or belief you would like to have.

For example, after you tap on feeling nervous about the speech next week, you could do a round of tapping on "Even though I was really nervous about giving that talk next week, I now feel calm and confident." (You might then use "calm and confident" as your reminder phrase.)

After you have tapped to reduce a headache, you could do a round of tapping on "Even though I have had that headache for days, I now feel clear and focused." (Reminder phrase is "clear and focused.")

Case Study: Cigarette Addiction

I was working with a young man who wanted to quit smoking cigarettes. He had several beliefs that were limiting his ability to successfully quit. These included "My friends won't be happy if I quit," and "It won't last, as it never does." The strongest belief was related to his family and the fact that no one had been able to successfully quit, and this really influenced his own self-efficacy.

The setup statements we used included this one: "Even though I can't quit, as no one in my family has ever successfully quit, I accept I have this belief." He rated this belief as quite strong, a 9 out of 10 on the SUD.

He also believed it was his destiny to be a smoker, and this made him angry at himself (at least a 9 out of 10). This became the setup statement: "Even though I think it's my destiny to be a smoker, and this makes me angry, I accept this is how I feel right now."

These are some reminder phrases he used on the acupoints:

- "I can't quit."
- "No one in my family has ever quit."
- "It's my destiny."
- "I'm stuck with it."
- "I feel angry."

After tapping for several rounds on these beliefs, the young man became more open to the idea of quitting. He started to feel less angry, and more positive that perhaps quitting was possible. We weren't trying to find a solution at all, nor brainstorm different quitting strategies. We were just acknowledging the feelings he had and the strength of the beliefs that appeared to be a roadblock.

After more talking and tapping, the young man was feeling quite positive. His concern and worry about his friends was low on the SUD scale, and he began verbalizing that he didn't have to copy his family's patterns. We ended this session and scheduled a time in two weeks to talk again.

In the two weeks in between, the client answered the following questions in order to develop setup statements when we next came together:

- Identify problem times that trigger cravings/urges to smoke.

- How do you feel when you see other people smoking?

- How do you feel when you smell cigarettes?

- How often do you think/obsess about smoking?

- How do you feel about yourself being a smoker?

- How would you feel if someone took away your cigarettes?

- Picture yourself with only one cigarette for the week. How do you feel?

- Picture yourself having half a cigarette and leaving the rest—how do you feel?

- Picture yourself throwing a whole pack of cigarettes away. How do you feel?

When he returned he reported the feelings that arose from these questions included deprived, sad, lonely, and bored. These were included in setup statements, and we progressively worked through them with tapping rounds.

Another two weeks later the young man reported he had significantly cut back on his smoking, by at least half a pack on most days. He said he wasn't using any willpower; he just didn't have the desire to smoke.

The final stage of the process focused on imagining himself in the future as a nonsmoker. This actually made him feel very positive. He thought about being places where he couldn't smoke cigarettes at all (e.g., flying on an airplane, or in a restaurant), and we did some tapping on mild discomfort about this. He pictured himself not smoking for a whole day and did not have any anxiety about this. In fact he felt "free."

I heard from this young man about three months later. He said he had continued to smoke three or four cigarettes a day after our last session, but within the next week had several days when he didn't smoke at all. He was surprised to realize he actually just forgot to smoke!

Within another few weeks, the few remaining cigarettes that he did smoke always seemed to be in the morning with coffee. He recognized this and changed his routine to having a cold drink instead. Eventually he forgot about lighting up.

I asked how his friends and family had responded, as this had been a concern in the beginning. He laughed and said they hadn't really noticed at first, and didn't treat him any differently if they were smoking but he wasn't. When they finally realized he wasn't smoking anymore, several of them asked him to share how he did it, as they wanted to as well!

Of course he shared about tapping. Many years later he is still a nonsmoker and has not had any relapses, and several family members have learned tapping and also quit. It is always a feel-good story when multiple people benefit!

SO HOW DOES EFT WORK?

EFT appears to affect the amygdala (stress center in the brain) and hippocampus (memory center), both of which play a role in the decision process when you decide whether something is a threat. EFT has also been shown to lower cortisol levels, which is the stress hormone. Too much cortisol can result in lowered immune function and ultimately affect our physical health (e.g., fatigue illnesses). This will all be discussed in later chapters.

Stimulation of acupoints like those used in EFT is believed to send a signal to the limbic or emotion system in the body and reduce its arousal.[2] This is why you tend to feel calmer after tapping. It is also why some people yawn while tapping!

EFT can also decrease activity in the amygdala, which is part of the brain's arousal pathway.[3] And studies with long-term follow-up points are showing the changes last over time, so there may be changes in the brain's neural pathways over time.[4]

So, ultimately, we have this stress-management tool—a way of calming the body and brain. This may then allow for clearer thoughts and better decision making.

In the case study of the young man tapping on his beliefs and feelings about quitting cigarette smoking, we mostly focused on how he *felt*. By tapping on anxious feelings about being with friends or family if he didn't smoke, and his anger that he wouldn't be able to stay quit (because the family couldn't), he was able to feel calmer.

It was then that he started to think of options that might help him quit. We didn't tap on new and innovative ways to quit cigarettes; we just tapped on the distressing feelings to help him reach a calm state. When his stress levels were low, he was more creative in his thinking.

In early sessions we did tap on the craving feeling he had in the mornings or during a scheduled break at work when everyone else smoked. (This is covered in Chapters 7 and 9.) When the amygdala is calm, the physiological response of a craving (chocolate, cigarettes, alcohol, and more) diminishes. This is why he reported he forgot to smoke as much and wasn't using any willpower.

Every session focused on being very specific to his own experience and paying attention to *exactly* how he felt or what he was thinking. This is a key ingredient in the success of EFT, and it is addressed next.

THE IMPORTANCE OF BEING SPECIFIC

Tapping works best when you are very specific. Tapping on great big global statements such as "I always run late" may not result in much change to your behavior. It is better to pick exact memories of running late and tap on what happened and how you felt.

Pick the earliest possible memory you have, as this may be closer to the origin of the behavior/pattern. You can also try to remember ever learning a behavior/pattern when you were quite young (e.g., by watching a family member). You may have feelings/beliefs that you adopted by watching someone else, rather than ever experiencing it yourself (the mirror neuron section below explains why this might happen). You can still tap on those times where you learned a pattern or behavior by watching someone else.

ASPECTS

When we tap on a situation, event, or memory that has caused us some distress, we often look for aspects. These are the parts of an event or memory that can include sounds, taste, smell, feelings, physical sensations, and thoughts or beliefs. Each event may not have all of these present, but it is important to look for them while tapping.

A fear of flying may include the following aspects:

- The fear of turbulence or loss of control
- The fear of aircraft or pilot failure
- The fear of terrorism
- The fear of tight spaces (claustrophobia)
- The fear of heights
- The fear of the unknown
- A past memory of flying where something went wrong
- Family stories of other people flying where something went wrong
- Physical anxiousness and other body sensations
- Blank mind or dazed thinking
- Emotions of terror and intense fear and thoughts of death

A food craving could also have many aspects:

- Smell of the food

- Taste of the food in your mouth

- Feeling in body/mouth as you eat the food (e.g., salivation)

- Past memories of that food or something similar

- General memories of food that are very positive and emotional

- Sight/vision of that food

- Sound of food when unwrapping it

As described, aspects could be a thought, a feeling, a body sensation, a sound, a smell, and anything else you think of. We think of them as jigsaw puzzle pieces that all come together to make up a state or memory. In a distressing moment, they tend to all blend together, and it can become harder to remember what actually happened.

However, tapping does help tease them apart, and sometimes you begin to become aware of different aspects while tapping. When someone smells something in their current life or hears a sound and is transported back in time to a memory, this might be an aspect from that original memory. They can have the same feelings now in their present moment as they did back then. (This is discussed with PTSD in Chapter 4 as it can be debilitating if the memory is disturbing.) The trigger for that smell or sound transports someone back in time, because it was stored as an aspect a long time ago.

Many aspects may need to be tapped on for an issue to be resolved. However, it may not take that long. EFT can work so quickly that it takes your breath away. Let's look at how this can happen.

TABLETOPS AND TABLE LEGS

We often use an analogy of a table when discussing how EFT can work quickly. The tabletop in the analogy often represents a global issue in life, and the legs of the table represent the times in life that reinforced that issue. Each of the legs and memories will have its own aspects.

Let's consider a common pattern of behavior: procrastination. Imagine someone who just does this all the time. Even when they try to be organized and efficient, they slip into a pattern of procrastinating.

In this example the tabletop is procrastination. It is the big global issue, and tapping just on "procrastination" may not change the behavior. The legs of the table are the events, memories, and times in that person's life where they *did* procrastinate; and some of these will be more significant than others (e.g., if there was a negative consequence from procrastinating, it may have been more impactful).

Tapping on all those specific events with all the aspects will be important. However, you may not have to tap on every single time in your life you ever procrastinated. (You may sigh in relief here!) It only appears important to tap on the *really significant memories* you recall about the topic. The procrastination table here will collapse when the largest legs are removed. The table will fall over even when several legs remain.

Figure 1C offers a visual example of a tabletop of someone who believes they aren't good enough. You can see the legs of the table include examples of specific times in their life where they haven't measured up (and each of these can have its own legs too). The idea is to tap on these individual memories (legs) as you become aware of them, and over time the belief of "I am not good enough" will change, and you will have a different reality. Chances are, you won't have to tap on every single memory.

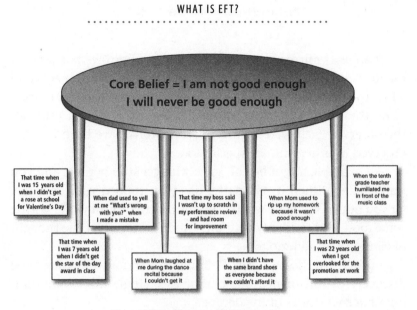

Figure 1C: Tabletop and table legs example

BORROWED BENEFITS IN EFT

Something unique occurs when watching other people tap, and we term this "borrowed benefits." This refers to the idea that simply watching someone else do tapping on their issues, while tapping along with them, can help you reduce the emotional intensity of your own issues. How can this be?

Dr. Jack Rowe, while a professor at Texas A&M University, was the first to notice this in a three-day EFT workshop for 102 people.[5] Participants completed a psychological symptom checklist one month prior to the workshop, immediately before starting, at one month afterward, and at six months afterward. There were no immediate changes; but at one and six months later, they had improved dramatically, even though they had been watching the sessions performed onstage. Their global psychological distress ratings improvements were maintained at the six-month mark.

It appears mirror neurons might explain borrowed benefits. A mirror neuron is a neuron that fires both when a person acts and when the person observes the same action performed by another. Thus, the neuron "mirrors" the behavior of the other, as though the observer itself were acting. Such neurons have been directly observed in other primate species too.

An example might be you see a stranger stub her toe, and you immediately flinch in sympathy like you stubbed your own toe. Or you notice someone wrinkle up his face in disgust while tasting some food, and suddenly your own stomach recoils at the thought of eating that food too.

In fact, psychologist Dr. V. S. Ramachandran has called the discovery of mirror neurons one of the "single most important unpublicized stories of the decade."

So the take-home message is that if you are tapping with someone (i.e., as a practitioner), it may be that anything in your own life that resonates with their story may also improve as you tap with them.

IDEAS FOR TAPPING WHEN YOU THINK OF A MEMORY: THE MOVIE TECHNIQUE

The importance of past memories and events in tapping is becoming clear. They form part of the experience you currently have. So we do look for them while tapping. You may be aware of them at the start of tapping, but other times as you are tapping, a fleeting thought passes through your mind, sometimes related, sometimes unrelated. Often this is part of your unconscious mind letting you know about a memory that may be important.

The process outlined next is called the Movie Technique and is one way to use tapping for past memories. Here are the steps.

1. Imagine the movie or memory and first give it a title. Make this title something fairly neutral, such as "The Day That Thing Happened." This allows you to

have some distance from it if it is distressing. Then give the movie title a SUD rating out of 10 (10: most distress, and 0: complete calm or neutral). Tap with the standard technique just for that SUD on the movie title until it feels lower in intensity before moving to step two.

2. After the SUD rating on the title of the memory feels like a 0 or 1, you are going to begin thinking about that past event as a movie. You can close your eyes for this or keep them open if you prefer to just stare at a spot ahead as you imagine in your mind's eye. You will want to imagine the memory is on a movie screen and you are watching it from the seats, or even the projection box, in a movie theater. It is important that you are watching yourself in the movie at a younger age. At no point are you in the movie yourself—you are *always* watching it from a distance. Chose a neutral point in time to be the starting point for the movie, before anything happened in the memory. This might be an hour before it happened, or even the day prior.

3. Play the movie memory very slowly from the neutral point, and stop the movie when you notice any negative or distressing sensation, thought, or anything else comes up. At this point freeze the movie and give that intensity a SUD rating out of 10. You might open your eyes at this point.

4. Use the standard steps: say your setup statement for that feeling, and tap until the SUD rating is a 0 or 1. When you feel calm for that first feeling, close your eyes again and rewind the movie memory to the beginning. Play it from the neutral start point in your mind, and check if that initial feeling is still low in intensity. If it is, continue playing the movie until you notice another concern. Remember this could be a thought, feeling, or body sensation. Stop the movie and do the same process as above. Rate the level of

intensity out of 10, form a setup statement, and tap through the points for as many rounds as you need until the intensity is a 0 or 1. If the first feeling you tapped on still seems high on the SUD scale when you check the movie, continue to tap on that before moving forward in the movie. Sometimes there is a different aspect that needs to be addressed before you feel truly calm.

5. Continue the same process of stopping the movie when you notice any intensity, using a setup statement to acknowledge it, and tapping through the eight points until the SUD is a 0 or 1. Eventually, you will be able to watch the whole movie in the theater, in your mind's eye, and feel neutral or calm about it. Sometimes people describe feeling more distance between themselves and the movie, and while it still happened in the past, they have more perspective now.

The Movie Technique doesn't change that the memory happened to you—but it does release any emotional charge that still might be in there.

If you feel distressed while doing this technique, the important thing is to *keep tapping.* It is the tapping process that calms the limbic system and will help you feel relaxed (and stop crying). However, if distressing memories come to mind and are overwhelming, it is always strongly recommended you engage with a professionally trained EFT practitioner to support you in processing them.

FREQUENTLY ASKED QUESTIONS ABOUT TAPPING FOR BEGINNERS

Q: How soon can I tap on my own?

You can use the technique on your own as soon as you understand the concepts in this chapter. There's no need to delay using the technique. However, always know you can seek the assistance and support of professional practitioners too.

Q: I worry about getting the setup or the tapping wrong. Does EFT have to be done precisely and perfectly?

No, there is no such thing as perfect EFT. For example, people with significant brain injury have reported benefits from doing their version of EFT that differed somewhat from what they were taught.[6] What mattered was that they were able to grasp the EFT concept; and because their unconscious brain understood the intention, they were able to gain benefits from the way they did it.

If you are really worried about getting it right (and without the help of a professional), tap with the setup statement "Even though I am worried about getting the words wrong, and it might not work, I accept myself anyway" (reminder phrase would be "worried").

Q: Can I make things worse if I don't tap exactly as taught?

No, you won't make anything worse—just stick to the basic steps. If you don't feel you completed the process because you haven't reached a SUD of 0 or 1, return to it another time. It is always best to tap until you feel calm, or there may still be aspects to deal with. Seek the support of a certified EFT practitioner if you do need assistance.

Q: I'm not sure I'm tapping in the right places. Will it matter if I don't get the exact point?

No, don't be concerned about getting the exact point. Using two or more fingers may give a better coverage of the points.

You can also purchase detectors or pens that measure electrical resistance of the skin to accurately locate acupoints of the human body. When you scan your body with the acupoint pen, it emits an acoustic signal to indicate the exact location. This technique enables even lay people to locate the relevant points.

Q: If I miss a point, will it affect the round?

No, you won't affect the round if you miss a point every now and then. If you wish, you can always go back to a missed point and tap on it.

Q: Do I have to use the same reminder phrase for each point in a round?

It helps to use the same phrase when you start using the technique and for the first few rounds; but as soon as you feel some confidence, you can change the reminder phrase. You may find that it changes naturally. Go with the new thought/feeling if one comes up.

Q: How do I know what feeling to tap for?

Whatever the main unwanted feeling is in that moment is the one you set up and tap for.

Q: Can I swap hands when tapping?

Yes you can use either hand, or even both. Some people like to use both hands while tapping, so both sides of the face and body are tapped at the same time. You don't have to do this, though. All the research trials only use one side of the body.

Q: What if there are so many feelings that I just feel confused or overwhelmed?

Rate, set up, and tap for feeling confused or overwhelmed. Just start there.

Q: What do I do if a different strong feeling (maybe associated with a thought or memory) comes up while I'm tapping?

Finish the round for the setup statement you started. Then immediately rate the new feeling/memory/thought, do a setup, and tap for that. The way to tap for a memory is outlined in the Movie Technique.

Q: If I'm in a situation where I feel uncomfortable saying the setup and reminder phrases aloud, can I say them to myself?

Yes, this still works. If you find yourself drifting and not staying focused, you may wish to continue at another time when you can say them out loud again.

Q: If I'm in a situation where I feel embarrassed or uncomfortable tapping, what should I do?

You can tap inconspicuously on any points you can and leave the others until you have the opportunity to tap in private. Also, consider tapping on the feeling of being embarrassed or uncomfortable in the situations concerned.

Q: If I don't have a particular feeling and I say the setup statement and tap with someone who does, will that give me the unwanted feeling?

No, you won't take on someone else's discomfort. Tapping with someone else for his or her discomfort can give you an awareness of a similar aspect that you may have. In that way you may get "borrowed benefits" from tapping with them and reduce your own discomfort.

Now that we've learned the basics of EFT, let's discuss the history of EFT and the different types (often called hybrids) that exist. Remember, the technique outlined in this chapter represents Clinical EFT, which is the version usually tested in research trials.

EFT BACKGROUND
AND HISTORY

The origins of tapping techniques lie in ancient Chinese medicine, specifically with the development of acupuncture. Acupuncture is a healing system that uses fine needles inserted in the skin at specific points along what are considered to be lines of energy, or meridians.[1] (When points are stimulated using pressure rather than needles, it is often referred to as acupressure.) In this approach, the flow of these energies underlies health and illness, and the stimulation of specific acupuncture points can enhance the flow of energy in ways that facilitate healing.

In Western medicine, acupuncture is most often used for pain management, as a complement to anesthesia, or in order to increase patients' comfort before and after surgery.[2,3] However, the method has been found to be effective in the treatment of a broad range of physical and mental ailments.

The 2017 Acupuncture Evidence Project drew on two prior comprehensive literature reviews: one conducted for the Australian Department of Veterans' Affairs in 2010; the other conducted for the United States Department of Veterans Affairs in 2013.[4] They evaluated existing studies using the Australian National Health and

Medical Research Council (NHMRC) levels of evidence criteria and the Cochrane GRADE system for assessing risk of study bias.[5,6] The aim was to present the current state of evidence and determine how the quality and quantity had changed from 2005 to 2016.

Of the 122 medical and psychiatric conditions reviewed across 14 broad clinical areas, research supported the effectiveness of acupuncture for 117 of them, with the evidence for 46 of them being at "moderate or high quality." Only 5 of the 122 conditions were rated at "no evidence of effect." An important trend identified in the review was that the level of evidence increased for 24 conditions during the 11-year period being investigated.[7] (Please refer to the Endnotes for the full paper and the conditions examined.)

In short, our most contemporary scientific evidence supports the effectiveness of the ancient healing system of acupuncture. So how did tapping on acupoints to treat psychological problems emerge?

THOUGHT FIELD THERAPY (TFT)

Dr. George Goodheart, an American chiropractor, appears to be the first Westerner involved in the use of modern tapping methods. (Tapping can, however, be found within acupressure which, like acupuncture, extends back at least 5,000 years.) Goodheart had been intrigued by acupuncture in the 1960s and introduced a variation into his own work as part of a new method he was developing, called applied kinesiology, which uses "muscle testing" to determine how the energies in the meridians are flowing and whether a particular intervention was effective.

Goodheart substituted manual pressure for the acupuncture needles by "percussing" (tapping) on the acupoints and observed benefits that were equivalent to those of acupuncture. Because of the nonthreatening and noninvasive nature of his techniques, Goodheart found that his patients were very open to this.

Fast forward to the 1970s. An Australian psychiatrist, Dr. John Diamond, created a variation of Goodheart's method and termed it "behavioral kinesiology." Diamond had his patients use affirmations (positive self-statements or thoughts) for emotional problems at the same time they tapped on selected acupoints.

In the early 1980s, American psychologist Dr. Roger Callahan studied applied kinesiology and learned about the acupuncture meridian system. He learned to apply this knowledge in the treatment of psychological conditions such as anxiety disorders and phobias.

Callahan stumbled upon these discoveries after working for two years with a patient, "Mary," who had an overwhelming fear of water. (She could not even get into a bathtub without having an anxiety attack.) Callahan had a home office with a pool that Mary had to walk by to get to the office, so she was already activated by the time each session began. One day, after she described the nausea and fearful feeling in her stomach, and with nothing so far having helped her, Callahan asked her to tap on an acupoint that is located directly beneath the eye. This point is, according to traditional acupuncture, linked to the stomach meridian. It felt like a long shot to him, but he thought that perhaps it would help calm the nausea and stomach discomfort.

But something remarkable happened. After tapping on this point for a while, Mary announced that her fear of water was gone. She ran outside to the swimming pool and splashed water on her face. She had never voluntarily gone near a swimming pool before. It appeared that tapping on the stomach point while thinking and talking about her fear of water had eliminated it. Over 30 years later, Mary reported that she was still free of this phobia.

Callahan continued to apply tapping while patients simultaneously focused on the problem at hand. He started to use different sequences of acupoints for different emotional problems, eventually developing prescribed tapping sequences (which he called "algorithms") for specific conditions.

This method was eventually called Thought Field Therapy (TFT), and it included muscle testing. Studies investigating this early form of tapping to overcome psychological problems have been impressive and are presented in Chapter 10.

ENTER THE EMOTIONAL FREEDOM TECHNIQUES (EFT)

Some of Callahan's early students wondered if a single algorithm might work as well as the customized sequences for different problems, a sort of "one size fits all" approach. It turned out it did.

After training with Callahan, Gary Craig, a Stanford-trained engineer who had become a personal performance coach, developed EFT, which as we've seen, uses a single set of tapping points regardless of the condition. This single-algorithm method has now become the most known tapping protocol and is the format that has been used in the majority of the clinical trials that have investigated tapping approaches.

In 1995, Craig assembled and released his first training video set, titled *The EFT Course* and the still-famous guide for the general public, *The EFT Manual*.[8] By the time Craig announced his retirement in 2010, this free guide to EFT had been downloaded in its English version more than two million times and was available in 20 other languages. Craig also taught his streamlined method in public workshops, making it his life's mission to share the technique with the world. After his retirement, he contributed the trademarked names EFT and Emotional Freedom Techniques to the public domain.

At the time of Craig's retirement, Dr. Dawson Church created EFT Universe, which is a large EFT training and certification program. Church is the author of the best-selling, award-winning science book *The Genie in Your Genes*, as well as the latest edition of *The EFT Manual*.[9] EFT International is one of the other major education, training, and professional development associations dedicated to advancing EFT.

SIMILARITIES AND DIFFERENCES OF TFT AND EFT

While their protocols diverge in many ways, TFT and EFT also share some key features. Both techniques involve tapping on specific acupoints while focusing on a targeted emotion or problem. The acupoints used by both techniques overlap considerably.

However, TFT uses only a subset of these points, with a specified sequence (the algorithm) for each of the problem categories it can address (such as anger, guilt, anxiety, depression), whereas EFT uses all of its tapping points for every problem. Despite this and other differences in their procedures, the outcome research shows both approaches to be unusually rapid and effective. That acupoint tapping is the distinguishing feature shared by both methods gives support to the position that acupoint tapping enhances clinical outcomes. The following chapter provides an overview of the EFT research. Chapter 10 examines the studies investigating TFT.

A NOTE ON THE DIFFERENT TYPES OF TAPPING

A quick Internet search on acupoint tapping or energy tapping will bring up hundreds of sites. You will also find many variations of tapping and hundreds of books on Amazon. It is not so unusual for a self-help approach to strike a popular chord and generate a great deal of notice and interest. The acceptance of a therapeutic innovation by the clinical and scientific communities, however, requires credible evidence and research.

While many hybrids or variations of EFT can be found, the term *Clinical EFT* has emerged to refer to the EFT tapping protocols that have been validated by research, along with the knowledge base that has developed from investigations of these procedures in the treatment of various populations and conditions.

The standards for the studies that comprise Clinical EFT are patterned after criteria originally developed by the American Psychological Association (APA) Division 12 Task Force on Empirically Validated Treatments.[10] One of the seven essential criteria is that the method be described in a written manual. Clinical EFT is based on the method defined in *The EFT Manual*, and most of the published EFT research has been guided by the manual. By defining a therapeutic modality according to a uniform set of procedures, researchers can be assured that conclusions from a series of studies are based on meaningful comparisons. That the techniques delivered in a study match what is prescribed in the manual is called "fidelity of treatment" and is essential for research within an emerging area of clinical practice.

As a researcher and academic, I am often asked to conduct research trials to test the effectiveness of variations of Clinical EFT. I usually decline, and for a very good reason in terms of the emergence of EFT as a field. As with any new approach, a foundation needs to be established. If the academic and general community are to accept the efficacy and mechanisms of an original method, precise or even accurate conclusions can't be reached if the evidence mixes apples and oranges.

In Chapters 3 through 9, the research we will explore is generally based on Clinical EFT. Not every study that has ever been published will be considered, but I will make recommendations of how to find research repositories should you wish to delve further. Chapter 10 looks at the evidence examining several other tapping techniques, including TFT. While relatively little research exists for EFT's variations and hybrids, I look forward to the day when the evidence for Clinical EFT has become so mainstream that we can shift our sights to innovations within this major clinical advance.

Chapter
3

THE MOUNTING
EVIDENCE

The sweepstakes question for the psychotherapy field is "Which therapy works best?" Opinions differ vehemently, with most therapists understandably strongly favoring the approach they use. Research evidence has not provided a decisive answer. Recognizing this deadlock way back in 1936, the American psychologist Saul Rosenzweig used the phrase "the Dodo Bird Verdict," after Lewis Carroll's *Alice's Adventures in Wonderland* character who declared, following a race, "*Everybody* has won, and all must have prizes."

Rosenzweig was proposing that all therapies are about equal in their effectiveness. His belief was that the common factors among therapies—the therapist's attention and caring, the focus on solving the patient's problems, and so on—had far more impact than the differences among the approaches. Rosenzweig's tongue-in-cheek Dodo Bird Verdict is that all therapies are winners, producing roughly equivalent positive outcomes.

This conclusion is still held by many researchers. A review of more than 200 studies, published in 1997, gave it further support.[1] While the paper established that psychotherapy is clearly better than no treatment, it found that when psychotherapies that are

31

based on sound principles were delivered by appropriately trained clinicians, they all worked about as well as one another. This conclusion was based on a meta-analysis, a statistical tool for drawing valid inferences from a large body of data, so it carried more weight than just the author's opinion.

If all therapies are about equal, however, why have more than 500 approaches to psychotherapy emerged?[2] Why are most clinicians convinced their methods work better than others? Why, for that matter, would psychotherapy not still follow Freud's original methods?

The psychologist who did the research that supports the Dodo Bird Verdict, Bruce Wampold, has thought deeply about this fundamental question, framing it in an influential book called *The Great Psychotherapy Debate*.[3] He identified three factors that are shared and common to all successful psychotherapies:

1. The therapist and the client have a strong bond and effective working relationship (often termed the therapeutic relationship).

2. The therapist and client both have an expectation that therapy will be successful.

3. The therapy approach includes the client engaging in health-promoting, beneficial actions.

It is around this third point that the debate about the relative effectiveness of different types of therapies hangs. Basically, does one set of meaningful "health-promoting actions" have greater impact than another? Or does the Dodo Bird Verdict stand as long as all three elements of successful psychotherapy have been properly implemented, as Wampold's study suggests?

ARE ALL THERAPIES CREATED EQUAL?

When in our Introduction I described EFT as representing a fourth wave in the evolution of psychotherapy, I was basing that bold claim on the power that stimulating acupoints has demonstrated for quickly changing brain activity. This is the "beneficial action" that the first-, second-, and third-wave therapies cannot do as well. The research comparing EFT with other approaches is still in a very early stage, so we can't definitively say that if Wampold's meta-analysis had included tapping therapies the results would have shown that, in fact, not all therapies are equal. But we have quite a bit of evidence suggesting that therapies that incorporate acupoint tapping have a distinct advantage over the ones that were included in Wampold's study. The Dodo Bird Verdict may not hold up with fourth-wave therapies.

EFT enjoys three features that distinguish it as a fourth-wave therapy: It is a true mind-body approach in that it includes direct interventions at the level of the body; it changes brain activity very rapidly; and it has special advantages in quickly and permanently shifting outdated emotional learnings.[4] Let's look at these features in depth.

- **A Somatic Intervention.** Therapists who are effective in working with people who have been traumatized have long recognized that talk therapies are not enough for healing the damage that is caused by abuse and catastrophe. The title of an influential paper and subsequent book, *The Body Keeps the Score*, by Dr. Bessel van der Kolk underlines this point. The physiological changes to the body and brain following trauma become "encoded in the viscera" and require treatments that "engage the safety system of the brain before trying to promote new ways of thinking." Effective therapies for severe trauma must address the body as well as the mind, and being able to do so is a great strength of somatic therapies.

  It is not just tapping on the skin that makes EFT a somatic intervention. Tapping initiates a cascading series of events in the brain and body that, as you will see below, impact hormone production, brain waves, blood flow within the brain, and gene expression in ways that enhance emotional health. And tapping has this impact not just for treating trauma but also in addressing everyday anxieties, upsets, and goals.

- **Rapid Results.** A decade-long research program at Harvard Medical School looking at what happens in the body when various acupoints are stimulated found that certain points almost instantly decrease the activation of the stress response in the brain. This research is described in more detail below, but suffice it to say that with elevated stress responses being part of many emotional disorders, the capacity to rapidly reduce them is a cornerstone in the speed and effectiveness of EFT. You will also see that EFT seems to require fewer sessions than more conventional therapies for equivalent outcomes.

- **Enhanced Information Processing.** David Feinstein's paper "How Energy Psychology Changes Deep Emotional Learnings" builds on the way the speed with which tapping (a central feature of "energy psychology") sends deactivating signals to the brain.[5] This rapid response combines with the brain's capacity to reprogram itself through a process called "memory reconsolidation." The outcome is that unhealthy responses to triggers, such as to the tone of your boss's voice, can be rapidly and permanently eliminated. Because much of the human experience involves responding to what life presents, being able to make shifts that promote healthier emotional responses and behaviors helps in overcoming a broad spectrum of emotional problems and also helps you to live a more successful and fulfilling life.

These three qualities come together to make EFT unusually rapid and effective in comparison with first-, second-, and third-wave therapies. In the remainder of this chapter, we will look at the evidence suggesting that EFT excels in each of these three areas. I will also list the conditions and populations for which the clinical trials of EFT have been promising, discuss some of the controversies around EFT, look at one of them in depth (Is it the "tapping" that makes EFT effective, or is it other factors such as the therapeutic relationship or the client's belief that it will work?), and we will close with a primer for understanding the research that is presented in the remainder of the book.

EFT AS A SOMATIC THERAPY

Medical director of the Trauma Center, Massachusetts, past president of the International Society for Traumatic Stress Studies, and professor of psychiatry at Boston University School of Medicine, Dr. Bessel van der Kolk has been vocal in his criticism of the tenets of traditional psychotherapy.[6] And parallel to this, he has been a public advocate of somatic approaches. Indeed, the early neuroimaging studies of PTSD showed that during exposure to a traumatic script, there was decreased Broca's area functioning (the speech area of the brain) and increased activation of areas in the right hemisphere related to emotion. Van der Kolk proposed traumatized individuals would not be able to verbalize precisely what they were experiencing, particularly when they become emotionally aroused. They would be too hyper-aroused to communicate, let alone process anything. Simply put, perhaps talk therapy by itself, even in the context of a warm, supportive therapeutic relationship, isn't enough to reverse the profound physical and emotional conditions in people with a history of trauma.

According to Van der Kolk, making meaning of a traumatic experience is usually not enough to process it. People need to have experiences that directly *contradict* the traumatic states of emotional helplessness and physical paralysis. They need to reexperience the event without feeling helpless, and this is exactly what EFT does. It is part of a group of newer body-oriented therapies (another is Eye Movement Desensitization and Reprocessing, or

EMDR) that all seek to desensitize clients without requiring them to fully engage in a verbal reliving of the traumatic experience. And the results are remarkable. These somatic therapies are producing benefits that traditional insight-oriented therapies are not. While EFT has someone focus on the distress (even if that is a body sensation or a thought), it is the somatic aspect of tapping that creates the decrease in amygdala and cortisol activity, resulting in calm. This very state of calm is a contradictory state to that of distress or trauma.

Whatever has caused excess cortisol in the body (e.g., trauma or otherwise), the hormone elevation can lead to problems in concentration, blood-sugar imbalances, sleep issues, decreased muscle mass, higher blood pressure, lower immune function (which may mean you are susceptible to more head colds), and increased abdominal ("belly") fat. However, cortisol has been shown to quickly respond after EFT.

In one study, 83 adults were randomly assigned to either a single hour of EFT (this means they didn't get to choose the treatment option), a psychotherapy group receiving a supportive interview (SI), or a no treatment (NT) group who just rested.[7] All adults had their cortisol tested (measured in their saliva) immediately before and 30 minutes after the intervention.

The EFT group showed clinically and statistically significant improvements in anxiety (approximately 58 percent) and depression (49 percent improvement). They also reported an overall reduction in the severity of symptoms (by 50 percent) and the range of their symptoms (by 42 percent, $p=0.001$).

Now, there were no significant changes in cortisol levels between the group who received the supportive interview and the no treatment (resting) group, *but* the cortisol in the EFT group dropped by 24 percent, which was significant. You might recall that I said the treatment was only one hour, so the speed at which EFT works can be breathtaking. What else was quite extraordinary was that the improvements in mental-health symptoms after therapy were also reflected in the reduced levels of cortisol. This tells us that the mind and body are most definitely in tune and interconnected.

EFT and Claustrophobia

We have just begun to see research emerging about how EFT and somatic tapping changes the brain. A small study with four people with claustrophobia (the fear of being enclosed in a small space or room and having no escape) showed that along with reductions in anxiety symptoms, a 30-minute tapping session brought elevated theta brain wave levels down to those of four nonclinical control participants.[8] They also had significantly reduced anxiety scores.

A quick note on brain waves: We have five different types of electrical patterns or "brain waves": gamma, beta, alpha, theta, and delta. These can be observed with an EEG (an electroencephalograph), which was used in the study. Each electrical pattern serves a purpose to help us cope with various situations. Theta waves are involved in daydreaming and sleep that results in feeling truly restored. Too much theta activity may make people feel depressed, but it can also help improve intuition and creativity.

EFT and Trauma Symptoms

In 2004 researchers looked at EEG patterns after the tapping technique in 10 people who had been involved in car accidents and were still suffering trauma symptoms.[9] They were brain mapped at the start and also completed questionnaires about their anxiety, depression, and avoidance of driving behaviors. They all received two EFT sessions and completed the same assessments, including the brain mapping.

All of the participants reported positive change after the EFT sessions, although four showed negative or no change when their brains were scanned again. Those who did improve showed increased regulation of the sensory motor cortex, decreased right prefrontal cortex arousal, and more changes in the occipital area of the brain. The researchers did say they believed the people who improved were the ones who were more compliant with the treatment. This first brain mapping study did show EFT was capable of producing brain changes, albeit not in every person.

EFT and Food Cravings

Brain imaging is a powerful technique that is now enhancing neuroscience research. Two ways this is done is through functional magnetic resonance imaging (fMRI) and positron-emission tomography (PET) scans. Both of these have been investigated by Harvard Medical School for more than 10 years for acupuncture. Their experiments have consistently shown that needling acupoints results in decreases of activation in the amygdala, hippocampus, and other brain areas associated with fear and pain.[10,11]

We now have studies emerging using fMRI, which is widely used to map brain activity, that show brain change after EFT. (I have run one of them, and the scans are presented in Chapter 7.) Here is what happened: We had 15 obese adults in total; 10 were allocated to an EFT treatment, and 5 to a control group (where they received no intervention for their cravings). They were all scanned using fMRI before and after a four-week EFT treatment phase. While they were in the machine, we showed images of high-calorie food (e.g., chocolate cookies, burgers and fries, ice-cream sundaes) and recorded what parts of their brains activated.

After the four-week EFT treatment, all adults were scanned again, and we showed the same images of food to see if anything changed. We saw a significant decrease in the activation in the EFT participants; and in some of them, there was no activation at all! This was amazing even for us to see. The control group still had activation in the parts of the brain associated with reward and loss. Chapter 7 will explain more of what we did and also show you the scans.[12]

EFT and Gene Expression

Finally, EFT has been researched at a physiological level, including its effects on genes. A pilot study compared an hour-long EFT session with a placebo session (where subjects thought they were getting a treatment, but it did not have an active component) in four participants.[13] What this small study found was incredible. After the EFT session, differential expression in 72 genes associated with the suppression of cancer tumors, protection against ultraviolet radiation, regulation of type 2 diabetes insulin resistance, immunity from opportunistic infections, antiviral activity, synaptic connectivity between neurons, synthesis of both red and white blood cells, enhancement of male fertility, building white matter in the brain, metabolic regulation, neural plasticity, reinforcement of cell membranes, and the reduction of oxidative stress occurred. This was a profound outcome and the first of its kind in this field.

There has since been another study that examined the regulation of six genes associated with inflammation and immunity after EFT treatment.[14] In a study of 16 war veterans with PTSD who received 10 hour-long EFT sessions, interleukins, which are responsible for regulating our body's inflammation response, changed significantly in expression. And "good" genes associated with improved functioning of the immune system were also changed. There was also a significant association between improvement in the veterans' mental-health symptoms and positive changes in the expression of their genes related to stress hormones.

EFT and the Central Nervous System

Exciting EFT research has been conducted on heart rate variability and heart coherence, the circulatory system using resting pulse rate and blood pressure, the endocrine system using cortisol, and the immune system using salivary immunoglobulin A.[15]

All of this added up to being one extensive measurement of the central nervous system (CNS). The CNS controls most functions of the body and mind and consists of two parts: the brain and the spinal cord. So basically this study was looking at the impact of EFT on all of this. The study also looked at changes in the psychological symptoms of anxiety, depression, PTSD, pain, cravings, and happiness.

The 31 participants were attending a five-day workshop and being taught 16 modules of EFT in a group, with 12 hours of practice. All of those measurements mentioned were taken at the start and end of the workshop, and the participants reported reductions in these areas:

- Anxiety (39 percent)
- Depression (46 percent)
- PTSD (32 percent)
- Pain (66 percent)
- Food cravings (80 percent)

They also reported their happiness increased (by 13 percent) as did their immune system (by 61 percent). They also had significant improvements in their resting heart rate (by 8 percent), their stress hormone cortisol levels (by 49 percent), their systolic blood pressure (by 6 percent), and diastolic blood pressure (by 11 percent). Systolic blood pressure refers to the pressure inside your arteries when your heart is pumping; diastolic pressure is the pressure inside your arteries when your heart is resting between beats.

These were some impressive gains over the five days. A downward trend was observed for heart rate variability, along with an upward trend for heart coherence, suggesting an improvement in cardiovascular health and function. Although the trend was not statistically significant, the authors determined that an additional 13 participants would have impacted the statistical significance of those measurements. What was exciting was that 60 days later when the researchers followed up with the attendees, everyone indicated they had maintained the gains in their psychological symptom improvements.

The Need for Homework?

A common strategy in the gold standard cognitive and behavior therapies is utilizing homework assignments as a mechanism to produce and strengthen beneficial treatment outcomes. Practicing skills outside the therapy session for permanent and long-term change is deemed essential. Indeed, engaging in homework activities to produce positive therapy outcomes has been examined in meta-analyses and results indicate that greater compliance with homework is associated with more beneficial treatment outcomes.[16,17] The type of prescribed tasks might include frequency checklists, symptom records, self-reflective journals, and structured activities like exposure.

However, one of the top cited reasons for therapy failure in cognitive behavioral therapy is homework *noncompliance*.[18] In adult clients, the rates of nonadherence range from 20 to 50 percent.[19] If tasks outside the client session are integral to positive outcomes, this poses an enormous issue for the three conditions above to be met if clients don't follow through. It is not the aim here to present the reasons why people are noncompliant; and regardless of whether they are internally or externally driven, what is evident is that therapy outcomes appear seriously affected by this problematic issue.

As mentioned, EFT's somatic component is more than tapping on the skin. It results in changes in the brain, DNA expression, hormone production, brain waves, and blood flow; and is it remarkably swift. This somatic component is indeed a "health-promoting activity" that does not necessarily rely on homework tasks being completed outside the tapping session.

EFT PRODUCES RAPID RESULTS

A distinguishing feature of somatic psychotherapies is that they are believed to produce positive outcomes with relatively few sessions. While brief EFT treatment programs may not be appropriate for every condition, the reality is that they can often achieve outcomes very rapidly.

An initial review of 51 peer-reviewed papers investigating clinical outcomes following a tapping process identified 18 randomized controlled trials.[20] These were then critically evaluated for design quality, and the author Dr. David Feinstein reported they consistently demonstrated strong effect sizes and other positive statistical results that far exceeded chance. It was also noted these outcomes occurred after relatively few treatment sessions.

Since then, further randomized controlled trials have demonstrated that EFT effectively treats phobias and certain anxiety disorders in one session. Extraordinary outcomes have occurred with single sessions, including significant decreases in cortisol and normalization of the EEG frequencies associated with stress. While conditions such as complex comorbid PTSD are typically expected to take longer to respond, EFT has resulted in relief for some clients after a single session.[21] Several studies have also indicated substantial reduction in symptoms and often an absence of diagnosis for PTSD after six hours of EFT treatment.[22,23] Gold standard therapies usually recommend 12 to 18 sessions for conditions such as PTSD. When EFT achieves the same outcome in considerably fewer sessions, it begs the question whether all therapies are indeed equal.

Length and Results of EFT Treatment as Compared to Other Therapies

Many research trials have now compared EFT to traditional and gold standard approaches. Invariably, EFT treatments achieve similar or identical outcomes in fewer sessions.

A large-scale study of 5,000 patients seeking treatment for anxiety allocated patients to cognitive behavioral therapy (CBT) that included medication if needed or acupoint treatment (Thought Field Therapy, the EFT precursor) with no medication.[24] Complete remission was reported by 76 percent of the patients in the acupoint group and 51 percent of the CBT group (p < .0002). Some improvement to complete remission was reported by 90 percent of the patients in the acupoint group and 63 percent of the CBT group (p < .0002). Those 90 percent of acupoint patients improved *in an average of three sessions*, compared with an average of 15 sessions for the CBT patients.

A pilot study of test anxiety in university students compared EFT to a Wholistic Hybrid derived from EMDR and EFT (called WHEE) and CBT and found significant reductions in test anxiety were observed for all three treatments. However, more rapid benefits were observed in the experimental treatments (WHEE and EFT): both WHEE and EFT achieved *in two sessions* the same benefits CBT did in five, potentially suggesting EFT and WHEE to have more rapid treatment effects.[25] (This is discussed in more depth in Chapter 8.)

This does raise the question, how can EFT achieve these same results as other approaches in less time? The somatic aspect of tapping is the clear answer. I briefly mentioned that Harvard Medical School conducted research over a period of more than 10 years into the mechanisms of acupuncture.[26] It was these studies that indicated that stimulating selected acupoints sends deactivating signals to the amygdala. Harvard's studies included brain imaging and indicated that the stimulation of certain points with acupuncture needles consistently produced prominent decreases of activity in the amygdala, hippocampus, and other brain areas associated with fear. If someone is aroused or distressed and repeatedly engages in a somatic activity such as EFT while bringing that to mind, it sends a conflicting signal to the limbic areas. The stress response becomes permanently altered when a process such as tapping deactivates the emotional centers of the brain. This then results in a calm state during any recall of those previously distressing thoughts, which brings us to how this then lasts over time.

EFT AS A POWER TOOL FOR CHANGING
DEEP EMOTIONAL LEARNINGS

Based on a special facility for bringing about memory recon-solidation, a unique feature of EFT is that the benefits appear to last well into the future without further treatment. Typically, we might expect that when exposed to the same situation in the future (e.g., seeing a spider), we would have to engage in tapping again to send the deactivating signal back to the brain. Dr. Fein-stein has rightly proposed that the common belief among neuro-scientists has been that once a new learning is consolidated into long-term memory, it is permanently installed. It may respond to extinction training, for example, but ultimately it is always at risk of reactivation.[27]

However, new research on memory reconsolidation shows that despite a lifetime of deep emotional learnings, the brain has a mechanism for "updating existing learnings with new ones,"[28] and core beliefs from childhood can be modified, strengthened, changed, or even erased![29] Neural pathways appear able to change, and three conditions have been proposed to facilitate this process:

1. The emotional memory or learning must be vividly accessed.

2. The client must experience both the situation they want to change and the contrary. This is called a "juxtaposition experience."

3. The juxtaposition pairing must be repeated sev-eral times.

In EFT step 1 occurs when the person states their concern in the setup statement. Tapping often results in an expression of the problem at a thought, feeling, or body-sensation level. Historical contributions to the problem might come to mind as memories from the past, giving access to the root cause.

In step 2, the somatic tapping reduces the emotional distress, and the brain therefore experiences a contradictory situation. An image or thought that was previously distressing is now no longer felt this way, and thus the neural pathway maintaining the old learning appears transformed by the new experience.

Step 3, the repetition phase, is vital for the contradiction phase to become permanent. In EFT the repeated rounds of tapping serve to identify additional aspects of the issue and process historical contributions.

At no point is it suggested that tapping changes or erases any learnings. Nor does it transform what actually happened. But the deactivating signal it sends to the emotional centers of the brain allows someone to remember what happened without distress. And the research is indicating these changes last over time.

So it may actually be that not all therapies are created equally, and there is no dodo bird. But there is a fourth wave—and it could be a tsunami. Before discussing how best to understand the research, let's briefly consider the populations and conditions where EFT has been studied.

Populations that have been studied with EFT include:

- College students
- Veterans
- Pain patients
- Overweight adults
- Hospital patients
- Athletes
- Health-care workers
- Gifted students
- Chemotherapy patients
- Phobia sufferers

Disorders and conditions that have been studied with EFT:

- General anxiety
- Test anxiety

- Phobias

- Obsessive-compulsive disorder

- PTSD

- General trauma

- Stress

- Depression

- Addiction

- Pain, including fibromyalgia and tension headaches

- Frozen shoulder

- Psoriasis

- Insomnia

- Seizure disorders

- Sporting / athletic performance

- Learning disabilities / educational challenges

- Epigenetic and physiological functioning

- General psychological functioning

The American Psychological Association's Division 12 Task Force on Empirically Validated Treatments created standards for evaluating psychological therapies. While they have recently been revised, the standards that were in place while most of the tapping studies were conducted have been summarized and include these requirements:[30,31]

- That a sufficient sample size be used for statistically significant effects ($p < .05$ or better)

- That valid and reliable assessment tools be used to measure change

- That treatment samples are assessed or diagnosed by qualified clinicians

- That random allocation to the active treatment and a control condition be used

- That interviewers be blind to group assignment in studies using interviews for subject selection

- That treatment manuals are utilized, or in the case of simple treatments, full descriptions within the study are provided

- That sufficient information be included so the study's conclusions can be reviewed for appropriateness, including sample sizes, use of assessment tools that identify targeted outcomes, and the magnitude of statistical significance[32]

A paper published in 2014 by EFT researchers Dr. Dawson Church and colleagues found that more than half of the published EFT studies at the time met these criteria.[33]

The next chapters in this book will unpack several major areas where EFT has the most research and it will become evident how the trials met the criteria above. As mentioned, you can keep reading chapter by chapter or go straight to one that interests you and take in the outcomes. But for now, we had also better consider the major criticisms of EFT.

DIFFERENCES OF OPINION

Like any new kid on the block, the rise and investigation of EFT has resulted in many critics speaking out. And given that we are about to launch into the outcomes of the existing research, it is important to consider what they say.

Criticism itself is not unusual. After all, anything new may threaten a status quo. And EFT is different from traditional "talk therapies." It involves the somatic element of tapping on acupoints, which may not be seen as conventional at all. Most critics of EFT argue that any changes that occur in clinical trials are due to the relationship between the client and therapist (as mentioned early in this chapter), or other factors like the client's personality, or even the placebo effect.

Placebo, Latin for "I will please," refers to any medical treatment that has no active properties (e.g., a sugar pill). It doesn't have to be a pill, however; it can be any "dummy" treatment too. The *placebo effect* is the positive effect on a person's health (physical or psychological) experienced after taking a placebo. It is triggered by their *belief in the benefit* of the treatment and their expectation of feeling better. Placebos are often used in clinical trials for new treatments and are thought to evoke complex neurobiological reactions that include everything from increases in feel-good neurotransmitters, like endorphins and dopamine, to greater activity in certain brain regions linked to moods, emotional reactions, and insight.

So critics of EFT will point to this and say a person's expectations that EFT will work is why they improve. However, in the highest form of clinical trial (the randomized clinical trial), people are randomly allocated to a condition (EFT, a control group who receives no treatment, or a different therapy), and they aren't allowed to choose. So this eliminates the bias that might exist if they really want to learn EFT and then report it works.

Randomly allocating people guarantees that, on average, treatment groups will be well balanced and ensure an unbiased estimate of the treatment effect. It is usually done with a computer program so researchers are not involved in the decision process.

When randomized studies show significant outcomes, it's a strong indication that the treatment has worked, and works for groups of people. When a study is replicated by different researchers and still achieves the same or similar results, this too points to the idea that it is the *treatment* that has worked, not the therapist delivering it, nor anything related to the people in that group at that time.

Another area of criticism raised involves the actual acupoints and what is really the active ingredient in EFT. Is it the words that are used, or is it the tapping? Do these work just as well separately? There have been some studies that have attempted to explore these ideas, and they tend to address the issue of placebo as well.

Finally, there is what is called a "translational gap" where any new therapies take some time before they are considered standard care. The American Institute of Medicine (the Health and Medicine Division of the National Academies of Science, Engineering, and Medicine) says this takes about 17 years, and only 20 percent of new therapies are accepted in mainstream.[34]

Replication

One of the measures of solid research is when other independent researchers replicate a trial and achieve the same outcomes. Replication tends to follow exactly the same protocols as the original study; and if it achieves the same outcomes, this suggests that the original results were reliable and valid. In other words, it suggests that researcher bias is likely to not have been at play.

WHAT MAKES EFT WORK? THE COMPARISON STUDIES

Comparison studies are those that tease apart different aspects of a strategy, to see what the active ingredient really is. They will often substitute an active ingredient for the missing one, eliminating the possibility that the missing ingredient is contributing to the treatment outcome (through a placebo effect). With EFT, often critics are interested in sham acupoint treatment, and this is where these studies focus. The first comparison study done for EFT compared EFT points, sham points, and tapping on a doll, and also included a control group who did nothing.[35] There were 119 university students allocated to one of those four conditions, and all were assessed for fear and anxiety levels.

The authors reported significant reductions in self-reported fear for all three tapping groups but not the control group. They stated that any effect from EFT was due to distraction or desensitization, rather than acupoint tapping. But there were some issues.

In the sham-point and doll-tapping groups, the students used their forefinger to tap, which inadvertently stimulated an acupoint there. The groups were effective, but ultimately all were using acu-point stimulation. The authors did not use valid assessments in their measurements nor full randomization to the groups. In the EFT group, they used acupoints not even included in the standard process, and omitted others. It is difficult to draw any solid con-clusions about this study, but it did start the process.

The next study to compare the aspects of EFT randomized uni-versity students into an EFT group or a control group who received mindful breathing exercises instead of tapping.[36] The students who did EFT reported more significant increases in enjoyment, hope, and pride and more significant decreases in anger, anxiety, and shame than did the breathing control group. The only prob-lem with this study was that the mindful breathing control group did not use the EFT setup or reminder statements; so while the actual tapping was the major difference from the control group, it was not the only difference.

The next study involved 56 university students who were assessed for stress symptoms and randomly allocated to an EFT group or a control group who tapped on sham points.[37] The stu-dents in the EFT group reported a 39.3 percent reduction in stress symptoms, while the sham tapping group only reported an 8.1 percent decrease. While this study supported EFT, it was limited in that the stress questionnaire used had not been validated, and one of the investigators led both the experimental and control groups, possibly contaminating the results.

A 2015 study involved 126 school teachers (assessed for burn-out risk) and is possibly the most effective comparison study to date.[38] The authors used two different schools that were similar demographically, to minimize any contamination, and allocated the teachers to an EFT group or a control group who tapped on sham points on the body in an otherwise identical protocol. They were all asked to focus on situations that contributed to burnout and stress while tapping. The control group tapped on the left forearm, about an inch above the wrist, with the underside of the fingers of the open right hand. This was important because no finger points were used or unintentionally activated (as in the first study discussed). Everything else was identical.

The results showed the EFT group was superior to the sham points group on the three indicators of burnout being tracked (emotional exhaustion, depersonalization, and personal accomplishment). And it was statistically significant.

In 2018, a meta-analysis reviewed whether EFT's acupressure component (the actual tapping) was an active ingredient in the therapy's success.[39] Six studies that included 403 adults with diagnosed or self-identified psychological or physical symptoms were compared. The acupressure groups showed moderately stronger outcomes than controls, and the meta-analysis indicated that the acupressure component was an active ingredient. In other words, outcomes were not due solely to placebo, nonspecific effects of any therapy, or nonacupressure components.

So in summary, one comparison study did not use a reliable and valid assessment; another did not provide enough information to obtain an effect size (for clinical significance), one did not adhere to the manualized EFT protocol, and others did not randomize the groups. The one study that was well designed and executed actually showed EFT to be superior to sham points. There is of course a need for further studies given the nature and placement of acupoints on the body, but the 2018 meta-analysis has indicated the tapping aspect is indeed an active ingredient in the technique.

How to Understand the Research

Before diving into the research studies, this section highlights what those studies mean and exactly what they measure. You will notice apples are not always apples when it comes to research trials!

- Outcome studies: These usually compare two different groups of people with the same condition (e.g., lower back pain) and report what they were like before and after EFT. These are often called randomized controlled or clinical trials (RCTs) and are the gold standard of research.

- Clinical reports: Sometimes these present as a single case study (on a single person only) and typically investigate conditions not as common or populations that are rarer or harder to run larger trials on (e.g., epileptics or prisoners). In medical research it is very common to read single cases on new or innovative types of surgery.

- Review papers: These are often called meta-analyses and examine many studies in the one area (e.g., anxiety). These are considered to be very important in research because they combine the results of many studies. These papers often look for similar trends or outcomes in a single condition. They are usually an examination of a group of studies that have been published by different authors, unconnected to each other. This helps with bias.

Research studies tend to report whether an outcome is statistically significant. This means it describes whether any differences noticed between the groups being studied are "real" or whether they are simply due to chance. So this is an important point.

In statistics we often talk in terms of a "p" value. This describes the chance (probability) of seeing an outcome in two groups (who we assume are the same).

If it is unlikely that the difference in outcomes occurred by chance alone, the difference is pronounced "statistically significant." And this is what we look for in a study.

P-values range from 0 (no chance) to 1 (absolute certainty). So 0.5 means a 50 percent chance, and 0.05 means a 5 percent chance.

Most research (in many fields, not just psychology and social sciences) says a p-value of .05 is the borderline of statistical significance. If the p-value is under

.01, results are considered statistically significant, and if it's below .005 they are considered *highly statistically significant*.

So if I tell you that in one of my studies, a change in anxiety levels from when the participants started EFT treatment to 12 months later was $p < 0.001$, then that means there was a 99.9 percent chance that the reduction in anxiety would *not* have been there if EFT did not work. This is considered truly excellent in research, and happens to be true for an EFT study I did run.[40] From this finding, scientists would infer that the EFT treatment was indeed very effective for anxiety in that study.

So a p-value of .05 means there's a very good chance (95 percent) that the difference in a condition would *not* be observed if the treatment had no benefit whatsoever. It is a strange way of describing things because we always start from the premise there is no difference. That remaining 5 percent means there is a very small chance you are wrong with what you found.

It is important to acknowledge that different things affect whether or not we see statistical significance in a study. For example, the size of the group of people we are observing is important. If only a few people are studied, and there doesn't appear to be any significance in the results, then it is feasible to think it might become significant if the group was larger. So you will often read in a limitations section of a study that future research should increase the sample size.

Another reason we sometimes don't see any significance is that the condition or symptoms may not be severe enough in the beginning (e.g., someone may rate their depressive symptoms as mild, so therefore we don't see any shift in this). My suggestion is that when you don't see any statistical significance in a study, look for *why*.

Another option is to consider *clinical significance* too. This type of significance really tells us what the client thinks: do they say the treatment helped them to return to normal functioning? We don't just rely on their thoughts about the treatment—we measure it mathematically. We normally ask a person to rate certain symptoms they have (e.g., stress) and compare it to a score typical of the "normal" population. This assists with knowing whether a treatment results in them experiencing that symptom in a "normalized" way at the end.

Another common method of determining the clinical significance between two groups is to calculate the effect size. Jacob Cohen (American statistician and psychologist) stated a "small" effect size is one in which there is a real effect (something is really happening), but which you can only see through careful study. A "large" effect size is an effect that is big enough and consistent enough, that you may be able to see it "with the naked eye."[41]

For example, if you walk into a room full of people, you will probably be able to tell on average, whether the men were taller than the women. A large effect size is therefore one that is very substantial, and you can see it with your naked eye.

Cohen's Effect Sizes
d=0.2 is considered a small effect size,
d=0.5 represents a medium effect size
d=0.8 is a large effect size

But for now, the mathematics lesson is done!

TAKE-HOME POINTS

This chapter has outlined the rapid rise and investigation of EFT in the past 20 years. It is still considered a new and innovative approach to reducing stress, but the mounting evidence is pointing to this being an effective stress and mood regulation tool. The longevity of EFT (how long it lasts) is explored in the individual chapters on conditions and populations; long-term follow-up after a study ends is the real proof.

Many trials report that participants don't actually continue tapping after the trial ends (there will always be exceptions to this). Because follow-up measures often show benefits are maintained well beyond the end of treatment, it highlights the memory reconsolidation and neural changes that occur. The three proposed features that distinguish EFT as a fourth-wave therapy indicate it has the ability to quickly and permanently shift distressing and disturbing emotional leanings that may no longer be relevant.

Let's turn now to an area that has had numerous trials, and one which can be devastating for a sufferer: post-traumatic stress disorder. This is a thoroughly researched area in EFT, and the results speak for themselves as to how effectively EFT works to assist the population with this condition.

Chapter
4

EFT, TRAUMA, AND PTSD

Sinclair was 27 years old when she first presented for therapy. She had been diagnosed by a psychiatrist with PTSD and discussed a long history of sexual abuse by a family friend since the age of 13. During the years this happened, she was living with an extended family member, as her parents were not able to care for her. She did not disclose any information to any adult, but instead suffered in silence.

When she turned 19 years old, Sinclair moved away to attend college, and the abuse stopped. However, years of drug use and an eating disorder ensued, and then a pregnancy. A year prior to attending therapy and motivated by having her own child, Sinclair started legal proceedings to have her perpetrator jailed. A long court case, which resulted in many other young adults coming forward to say they too had been abused, finally ended and the perpetrator was sentenced.

Sinclair's level of distress, however, did not decrease as a result. The PTSD symptoms she dealt with daily included avoidance of any beaches (as this is where the abuse took place), hypervigilance, severe anxiety, frequent nightmares and profuse sweating, and social isolation.

She was able to process her traumas with EFT over a six-month period, and now has another child and is in a loving relationship. She describes that while those years of her life were horrific and should never have happened to any child, they are distant memories that have lost their emotional charge. She is able to talk of her perpetrator without fear and no longer meets diagnostic criteria for PTSD.

WHAT IS PTSD?

In order for someone to be diagnosed with PTSD, a trauma must have happened and symptoms present for at least a month. There are four major types of symptoms that occur for most people after a trauma: reexperiencing the trauma, avoidance of anything that reminds you of the trauma, arousal such as feeling on edge or not sleeping, and negative changes in beliefs and feelings.[1] Other criteria include duration of symptoms, functioning, and that symptoms are not attributable to a substance or co-occurring medical condition.[2]

PTSD can occur in anyone at all, in people of any age, ethnicity, nationality, or culture. PTSD affects approximately 3.5 percent of American adults, and an estimated 1 in 11 people will experience PTSD in their lifetime.[3] There is now also a preschool subtype of PTSD for children ages six years and younger.

While the definition of trauma is different for everyone, the traumatic events most often associated with PTSD for men are rape, combat exposure, childhood neglect, and childhood physical abuse. The most traumatic events for women tend to be rape, sexual molestation, physical attack, being threatened with a weapon, and childhood physical abuse.[4]

As you can see, a PTSD diagnosis can be very disabling for a sufferer and interfere with the most basic functioning. While some people may recover within a few months of a trauma, others can suffer for years.

There are a number of therapy options recommended for PTSD, and EFT as a proposition has been extensively examined. These investigations have demonstrated a substantial reduction in symptoms for sufferers, so let's have a look at the evidence across different areas.

PTSD IN VETERANS

An initial 2010 EFT study to develop a trauma protocol by Dr. Dawson Church focused on a five-day treatment program for 11 veterans and their family members.[5] They received follow-up 1, 3, and 12 months later as well. The results showed significant improvements in the measures of PTSD symptoms immediately after the five days, and none of the veterans scored in the clinical range for PTSD. The severity and breadth of their psychological distress decreased significantly, and most of the gains held over time. It was the first time EFT as a treatment was presented as being an effective intervention post-deployment.

An observational study of seven veterans (three males and four females) in the same year investigated psychological symptoms change in veterans after six one-hour sessions of EFT delivered over one week.[6] Two different practitioners delivered the EFT intervention, but it was a standardized form. While there was no active comparison group, and follow-up was only at three months, anxiety severity decreased significantly by 46 percent, depression by 49 percent, and PTSD by 50 percent. These gains were also maintained at three months.

In another study of a group of veterans meeting the clinical criteria for PTSD who were randomly assigned to either EFT treatment (30 in total) or standard care (29 in total), those who met the clinical criteria for PTSD and received the six-hour EFT intervention were found to have significant reductions in psychological distress and PTSD symptoms following EFT treatment. [7]

What was quite outstanding was that following both treatments, 90 percent of those who received EFT no longer met criteria for PTSD, compared to only 4 percent in the standard care group (i.e., 96 percent of the standard care group continued to meet the clinical criteria for PTSD following standard care). Three months later, 86 percent of those who received the EFT intervention remained in remission, while 80 percent remained in remission at six months. These results were consistent with other published reports showing EFT's efficacy in treating PTSD and comorbid symptoms and its long-term effects.

A 2016 study reported almost identical outcomes. A study of 58 veterans who scored 50 or greater on the military PTSD checklist (indicating clinical symptom levels) were randomized into a treatment as usual (TAU) group (26 veterans) or an experimental group (32 veterans).[8] The intervention group received six one-hour EFT sessions in addition to TAU. The EFT group showed a significant reduction in a PTSD score from 65 ± 8.1 to 34 ± 10.3, while those in the TAU group showed no significant change. The TAU group was then treated with EFT and both groups combined for analysis (this is common so that individuals in the former "waitlist" group still receive an intervention).

In the combined EFT group, post-treatment scores declined to an average of 34 (a decrease of 52 percent). The participants maintained these gains at three- and six-month follow-up, with an average six-month score of 34. Psychological conditions such as anxiety and depression also declined significantly, as did physiological markers of insomnia and pain. The study reported an effect size of Cohen's $d=3.44$, indicating a very large treatment effect.

In a similar vein, 218 male veterans and their spouses attended one of six weeklong retreats to learn EFT and other energy psychology methods (EFT was delivered in a single four-hour group session and then three one-hour individualized sessions).[9] At the end of the week, only 28 percent of veterans still scored in the clinical range for PTSD, and spouses (who had never before been measured in a study) also demonstrated substantial symptom reductions. At the start of the week, 29 percent of spouses met clinical criteria for PTSD, but at the end, only 4 percent did. The veterans maintained their gains four and six weeks later, and the PTSD symptom decreases also continued for the spouses.

It is important to note that the other options in the study that week included massage, yoga, Reiki, and acupuncture. Furthermore, everyone participated in a half-day equine-assisted therapy session and a Native American ceremony at the beginning and end of the retreat. All of these options may have also impacted the EFT outcomes and PTSD-symptom reduction.

In a recent 2016 study investigating subclinical PTSD symptoms as a risk factor for a later diagnosis, 21 veterans were tracked to see if they developed the disorder.[10] They were randomized into a treatment as usual (TAU) wait-list group and an experimental group, which received TAU plus six sessions of EFT. Symptoms at the start of treatment indicated a score of 39 ± 8.7 on the PTSD Checklist—Military Version (PCL-M), in which a score of 35 or higher indicates increased risk for PTSD. There were no differences between the two groups at the start. The TAU group had no changes during the waiting period and received the EFT treatment at the end of this period.

For the collapsed groups after treatment (because both ended up receiving EFT), there was an average score of 25, which indicated a 64 percent reduction. The veterans maintained their gains at three- and six-month follow-up, with an average score of 27. A Cohen's d=1.99 indicated a large treatment effect. This meant the differences between the veteran and the TAU groups would have been noticeable even to the layman. The study also showed reductions in traumatic brain injury symptoms and insomnia. The authors noted EFT may be protective against a later PTSD diagnosis.

COMPARISON OF METHOD OF DELIVERY

Does the delivery of the therapy matter? In one of the first studies to compare delivery of EFT via coaches versus licensed therapists, 59 veterans were randomly allocated to EFT treatment (30 veterans) or a wait-list control group (29 veterans).[11] It is important to note 149 veterans were approached for the treatment, and only those motivated may have volunteered. The participants received six sessions of EFT over a month, with 26 receiving it from a therapist and 33 from a coach. Measures of PTSD included a PTSD checklist and also a symptom-assessment questionnaire.

There was a significant decline in the percentage of veterans still meeting PTSD criteria after only three sessions of EFT: 47 percent still met it in the coach condition, while only 30 percent still met it in the therapist condition. However, improvements continued afterward; and at the six-session mark, only 17 percent of the coach condition and 10 percent of the therapist condition still met criteria. These gains were also maintained three months later. While the statistical differences between the coaches and therapists were nonsignificant, the therapist group did have lower levels of psychological distress at the end.

The method of delivery of EFT has been investigated with PTSD veteran sufferers, and a comparison of traditional face-to-face delivery versus telephone delivery showed positive outcomes.[12] Each group received six one-hour EFT sessions, which were manualized for standardization. In total, 24 veterans received telephone sessions, and 25 received face-to-face sessions. The telephone group improved significantly in PTSD symptoms after the six sessions, whereas the face-to-face group only took three sessions to achieve these gains.

After six months, 91 percent of the face-to-face group no longer met criteria for PTSD, but only 67 percent of those treated via telephone no longer met it. While there was no comparison treatment, and veterans self-selected to the two groups rather than being randomly allocated, telephone delivery was effective for two-thirds of patients. It suggested that for some it might be a viable alternative for those unable to attend face-to-face sessions.

COMPARISON OF EFT TO OTHER APPROACHES FOR PTSD

EFT has been compared to EMDR for PTSD in 46 adults (the U.S. Department of Veterans Affairs has accepted EMDR as a viable treatment for veterans with PTSD).[13] In this study the participants were randomly allocated to EFT or EMDR (23 in each), and results indicated *both* interventions produced significant outcomes at the end of treatment and three-month follow-up. While a slightly higher proportion of EMDR patients showed substantial clinical changes, the treatment effects were similar in both groups. Given EMDR is accepted as an evidence-based treatment, and EFT achieves similar outcomes in clinical trials, then it is a logical next step to consider EFT as a viable option.

An evaluation of EFT and Narrative exposure therapy (NET) as treatments for PTSD investigated 60 male Iraqi students who met the DSM-IV PTSD criteria and were aged between 16 and 19 years.[14] They were randomly divided into three groups, with 20 participants in each group. The EFT and NET groups received four therapy sessions each, while the control group received no treatment.

The EFT group reported a significant difference in all PTSD cluster symptoms, although the NET group only reported a significant difference in avoidance and reexperience (not hyperarousal). There were no significant differences between the groups relating to social support, coping strategies, and religious coping. These changes were maintained for the EFT group at 3-, 6- and 12-month follow-up; and the effect size of EFT was higher than NET and the control group, thus indicating that EFT was more effective than NET.

And finally, a 2015 publication reported on a comparison between cognitive behavioral therapy (CBT) and EFT for sexual gender-based violence (SGBV).[15] The study included 50 internally displaced female refugees who had been victims of SGBV in the Democratic Republic of Congo (DRC). They all received two two-and-a-half-hour treatment sessions per week for four consecutive weeks (eight sessions in total). The women indicated significant post-test improvement in both groups on measures of trauma, PTSD symptoms, and general mental health. They also maintained their gains whether treated with EFT or CBT, and overall demonstrated the effectiveness and non-inferiority of EFT to a gold standard intervention.

THE IMPORTANT REVIEWS

A systematic review assessing the evidence for 15 new or novel interventions for the treatment of PTSD found there were four interventions with moderate-quality evidence from mostly small- to moderate-sized randomized controlled trials.[16] One of the named interventions was EFT. The important thing about this study was it was led by an independent university with impartial researchers.

Another systematic review of seven studies investigating EFT in the treatment of PTSD found a very large treatment effect (weighted Cohen's d=2.96, 95 percent CI 1.96-3.97; p < 0.001) for the studies that compared EFT to usual care or a wait list. Remember, above 0.8 for Cohen's d indicates a large treatment effect, and this review found an effect of 2.96!

The authors used the APA standards as their quality-control criteria when selecting studies for inclusion, and also found that a series of 4 to 10 EFT sessions was an efficacious treatment with *no adverse effects* for PTSD with a variety of populations.[17] When we talk about the speed of EFT, this is precisely what we mean.

In 2017 Drs. Church and Feinstein reviewed all the Clinical EFT research to date for PTSD with a focus on veterans and service members. The published studies indicate that PTSD symptoms are typically improved in very few sessions—ranging from one session for a phobia to 4 to 10 sessions for PTSD. EFT is considered especially suitable for veterans and military for these seven reasons:[18]

1. The depth and breadth of treatment effects

2. The relatively brief time frames required for successful treatment

3. The low risk of adverse events

4. The minimal training time required for the approach to be applied effectively

5. The simultaneous reduction of physical and psychological symptoms

6. The utility and cost-effectiveness of Clinical EFT in a large-group format

7. The method's adaptability to online and telemedicine applications

TRAUMA

The application of EFT for general trauma outside of PTSD has also been studied.

Ten adults who had been in an auto accident (within the past year) and were continuing to suffer from reported moderate to severe traumatic stress received two sessions of EFT.[19] All clients had brain-wave assessments (using a quantitative electroencephalograph, qEEG) before and after EFT treatment. They also completed questionnaires relating to anxiety, depression, and avoidance of driving/riding in a motor vehicle. Everyone reported positive change immediately after the EFT treatment, but four reported no or negative changes at the time of the last brain assessment.

Those who reported the benefit of EFT had increased 13–15 Hz amplitude over the sensory motor cortex, decreased right frontal cortex arousal, and an increased 3–7 Hz / 16–25 Hz ratio in the occiput (back of the head). The authors hypothesized that the improved subjects may have been more compliant with treatment recommendations whereas the unimproved clients were not. This is not an uncommon phenomenon across many therapeutic modalities.

Following the 2010 Haitian earthquake, which did widespread damage, 77 male seminarians were assessed for PTSD.[20] The purpose of this study was to evaluate EFT delivery to a traumatized population, and 48 of the men (62 percent) exhibited scores in the clinical range for PTSD. While the study lacked a control group, after two days of EFT, not a single participant scored in the clinical range on the PTSD measure—this was an outstanding result. The average reduction of PTSD symptoms was 72 percent after the two days. The results were consistent with other studies and pointed to the potential of EFT for those experiencing natural disasters.

A project called "Change Is Possible" in the San Quentin State Prison in California has offered EFT to life-sentence and war-veteran inmates for some years. Prisoners generally receive five sessions of EFT from a trained practitioner, with a three-session supplement one month later.[21] Similarly, another study randomized 16 males (aged 12 to 17) from an institution to which juveniles were sent by court order. This was usually due to being physically or psychologically abused at home.[22] In this study the teens were assessed with a SUD rating and the Impact of Event Scale, which measures two components of PTSD: intrusive memories and avoidance symptoms.

One group was treated with a single session of EFT, and the wait-list control group received no treatment. Thirty days later, participants were reassessed and there was no improvement for the wait list, but posttest scores for the EFT group improved to the point where all were nonclinical on the total score, as well as the intrusive and avoidant symptom subscales and SUD ratings. This was an outstanding result and consistent with studies in adults. It again points to the impact EFT has after relatively few sessions.

THE MECHANISM OF CHANGE

So why does EFT actually work for PTSD and trauma? Dr. David Feinstein, clinical psychologist and an internationally recognized leader in the field of energy psychology, offers some reasons.[23] Dr. Feinstein suggests that combining the brief psychological exposure of EFT with the manual stimulation of acupoints integrates established clinical principles. In 2010 he reviewed two randomized controlled trials and six outcome studies with military veterans, disaster survivors, and other traumatized individuals, and suggested that tapping on selected acupoints during imaginal exposure *quickly and permanently* reduces maladaptive fear responses to traumatic memories and related cues.

At the time this was a controversial approach, and the speed at which EFT was working in this field was unheard of. Feinstein proposed deactivating signals were being sent directly to the amygdala (brain stress center), resulting in the rapid decrease of threat responses to things that were benign.

Furthering the memory reconsolidation proposal in Chapter 3, one of my own doctor of philosophy graduates Mahima Kalla (Monash University, Melbourne) also raised the notion that memory reconsolidation mechanisms may be utilized for therapeutic change in neuropsychiatric disorders such as PTSD and phobias.[24] Kalla wrote that maladaptive fear memories, usually attributed to Pavlovian associations, are considered to be at the crux of these disorders. This means fears become associated with benign or neutral things, as Pavlov famously linked food and the sound of a bell for his dogs by ringing it when feeding them. They eventually salivated with the sound of a bell ringing in the absence of any food being presented. If abuse happens to someone in a certain room, often a neutral item might set off the trauma response because it has become associated with the abuse (e.g., the color of a chair).

The memory reconsolidation theory suggests that upon retrieval, the trauma memories become labile (easy to change) for a few hours. During this time, expectancy violation or prediction error can induce memory destabilization and lead to therapeutic change. This particular article proposed that EFT can specifically be used to reconsolidate memory and therapeutic change. The EFT protocol combines three crucial elements of therapeutic change: retrieval of fear memories (the exposure aspect); incorporation of new emotional experiences and learnings into the memory, creating a prediction error (after the acupoint tapping); and finally reinforcement of the new learning (which we see in follow-up aspects of studies). This is commensurate with Feinstein's and others' suggestions and may not be as radical as originally believed.[25,26]

PRACTICAL TIPS FOR USING EFT FOR PTSD

In 2017, clinical best practice guidelines for the use of EFT to treat PTSD were proposed.[27] In a survey of 448 EFT practitioners, a "stepped care" treatment model used by the United Kingdom's National Institute for Health and Clinical Excellence (NICE) was used to inform guidelines. Most practitioners (63 percent) reported that even complex PTSD can be remediated in *10 or fewer EFT sessions*. Some 65 percent of practitioners found that more than 60 percent of PTSD clients are fully rehabilitated, and 89 percent stated that less than 10 percent of clients make little or no progress.

Based on this feedback, the authors recommended a stepped-care model, with 5 EFT therapy sessions for subclinical PTSD (when it doesn't quite meet full diagnosis) and 10 sessions for clinical PTSD, in addition to group therapy, online self-help resources, and social support.

Overview of the Clinical Guidelines

The authors suggested the risk of PTSD should be mitigated using a proactive approach to develop resiliency. In the NICE model, the patient is offered the least intrusive potentially effective intervention first. If the patient does not benefit, or prefers not to continue, the next step is offered. The NICE guidelines emphasize the importance of integrated care, because many mental-health conditions share similar neural pathways.

Step 1: Involves identification, assessment, psychoeducation, active monitoring, and referral for further assessment and interventions. NICE recommends using the PTSD Checklist (PCL); and in a military population, a score of 35 or greater indicates PTSD risk probability.[28] The PCL is a 20-item self-report measure that assesses the 20 symptoms of PTSD according to the Diagnostic and Statistical Manual of Mental Disorders (DSM-5). The PCL has a variety of purposes, including the following:

- screening individuals for PTSD
- making a provisional PTSD diagnosis
- monitoring symptom change during and after treatment

Step 2: NICE recommends treatment using Trauma-Focused Cognitive Behavioral Therapy (TF-CBT) or EMDR. These recommendations do not include EFT because most of the earlier referenced studies had not been published at the time the guidelines were developed. The authors of the clinical-practice guidelines for the use of EFT to treat PTSD have recommended an update of the guidelines based on currently published research.

When Clinical Scores are 35 to 49 in Initial Assessment

For subclinical scores (35 to 49) in the initial assessment (PCL), the EFT clinical guidelines recommend that treatment should be as usual, plus these steps:

1. Five individual EFT therapy sessions

2. One instructional session on using the BATTLE TAP interactive online coach

3. Three Borrowing Benefits group therapy sessions (If members of the client's family are willing and able to attend a Borrowing Benefits sessions, they should be invited.)

BATTLE TAP is an interactive virtual EFT–coaching software program, a "ready-to-use" adaptation of EFT created by founder Gary Craig.[29] Borrowing Benefits is the notion that simply watching someone else do EFT on their issues while tapping along with them can help you reduce the emotional intensity of your own issues (see Chapter 1).

Dr. Church and colleagues suggest that if symptoms are still above 34 (PCL score) when step 1 is complete, then three more sessions plus an additional BATTLE TAP instructional session be carried out. Three months after the final therapy session, if symptom levels are still above 34, monitoring the client and performing regular follow-up assessments are recommended.

When Clinical Scores Are > 49 in Initial Assessment

Treatment as usual should occur as well as these steps:

1. Ten individual EFT therapy sessions

2. Two sessions using BATTLE TAP

3. Five Borrowing Benefits group sessions (If members of the client's family are willing and able to attend Borrowing Benefits sessions, they should be invited.)

If symptom levels are persistently above 40 after the above has been conducted, then they recommend three more individual therapy sessions and an additional BATTLE TAP session, as well as five additional Borrowing Benefits group sessions.

Three months after the final therapy session, if clinical symptoms still persist, the authors recommend escalating intervention to steps 3 and 4 of the NICE guidelines, which advocate appropriate medication and intensive individual psychotherapy.

A Proactive Approach for Using EFT for Active-Duty Military

Dr. Church and colleagues in the above study also advocate for a proactive approach using psychoeducation and Borrowing Benefits to mitigate the risk of development of symptoms in active-duty military. This is a unique and potentially powerful approach. It has two arms:

- *Pre-deployment Component:* Independent of the PCL-M assessment, three days of group EFT training using Borrowing Benefits as stress-inoculation therapy, including an introduction to BATTLE TAP is recommended.

- *Post-deployment Component:* Independent of the PCL-M assessment, seven days of group EFT therapy using Borrowing Benefits and BATTLE TAP are recommended. Practitioners are to offer individual psychotherapy sessions if requested by active-duty military.

NOTES FROM A PRACTITIONER

Julie Vandermaat, a sexual assault counselor in Australia, shared this story with me of working with "Stella," a young Aboriginal woman. Stella was referred by her medical practitioner for PTSD, anxiety, and depression caused by childhood trauma. For years she had been going to appointments with psychologists and psychiatrists, and while she did everything suggested, her symptoms did not improve.

As a teenager Stella used to cut herself. She tried to kill herself and ended up in the mental-health inpatient unit a number of times. As time went on, she no longer wanted to end her life—all she wanted to do was feel better.

Julie was the last counselor Stella was going to try.

At her first appointment, Stella was so anxious she was visibly shaking. She explained it took her lots of courage to come to that first appointment. But she engaged very well and was able to talk about being exposed to a lot of violence and drug and alcohol abuse while growing up.

Stella explained she had been sexually assaulted a few times, but the worst trauma was being violently sexually assaulted by a trusted adult family member when she was a teenager. She reported this to the police, had a forensic medical examination, and the perpetrator was jailed. However, she was still traumatized.

Stella reported at the first session that she was barely leaving her house. She was "petrified" that the perpetrator or another family member could find her and hurt her. She was hypervigilant, and always kept her back to the wall. Her PTSD score was 47 out of 60 on the Child and Adolescent Trauma Screening questionnaire, and on the Hospital Anxiety and Depression Scale she scored 16 for anxiety (severe) and 11 for depression (moderate).

Her mood was 3 out of 10, and her sleep was terrible as she was startled by any noise. She never felt hungry, as she felt physically sick all the time. Stella explained that food triggered her to think about all the happy times and meals that used to be shared together in her big extended family.

But since the sexual assault, Stella lost most of that family support, as only a handful of family members believed and supported her when she reported the crime. Most people blamed her, or thought she lied. She also washed her hands 20 times an hour, as she always felt dirty. "I can't get myself clean," she said, and her hands were cracked and sore.

The first EFT session focused mainly on fear: that the abuse could happen again, or that the perpetrator or a family member might find her and hurt her. This was 10 out of 10 for Stella. Julie also focused on shame, feeling "dirty" and "not human" as these were also 10 out of 10 for Stella. In her body, Stella felt this mostly in her stomach, where she was constantly nauseated, and she described this feeling as black in color.

After the first EFT session, Stella was relaxed, laughing, and smiling and rated her feelings as 6 out of 10. When she left, Stella stated she felt more hopeful that maybe there was something that could help her. After that EFT session, she said she had "the best sleep ever," and was more able to eat without feeling so sick.

Stella explained at the second session that many of the thoughts were still there, but that she was able to just acknowledge them without getting caught up in them. She said, "I'm not letting the thoughts define me anymore."

The second session focused on "Am I normal?" and Stella was able to reframe her trauma. She said that through this experience, she was able to save her mother and herself from further exposure to drugs, violence, and sexual assault, which she felt was considered "normal" in the culture of her extended family.

By the third appointment, Stella reported her anxiety was much better, rating it as 4 out of 10 during the day, although still very high at night. Stella mentioned that after two sessions of EFT, she was finally able to relax enough to close her eyes in the shower, and this was something she hadn't done in years. She was very happy with the sessions. At the fourth appointment, her screening measures had not changed much, but her reflections were:

"I feel human now. I am as normal as I can be, considering what has happened to me."

"My life is not 'stuffed.' It has been affected, but I can live with it (the trauma) now and work through it."

"I am okay. I am not useless. I can help somebody else through sharing my experience, and that makes me feel good about myself and proud of myself."

Stella was only washing her hands about 20 times a day (not per hour). Her hands looked smooth, and the skin was healthy. She rated her shame feeling as 4 out of 10—which she said was "a normal part of being Aboriginal." (Julie felt very sad to hear this, but Stella was accepting of the situation.) She rated her general mood as 5 out of 10 and described a lot more self-love and self-acceptance. She said, "I am content with my body now."

Julie then asked Stella to join her to speak about EFT to a forum of youth mental-health professionals. It was an informal end-of-year meeting, focusing on "what has worked well in 2017." Stella was enthusiastic about the idea and said, "I am still anxious and nervous at times, but I know I am safe."

Stella spoke beautifully at the forum, and the audience was stunned. She talked about how she liked EFT as it felt safe and gentle. She described feeling in control of the process while she is tapping. Stella also appreciated that she decides what the sessions focus on. She said she has found more hope through a few sessions of EFT than she has in years of traditional talk therapy, which inspired her to want to share her journey to help others who have experienced similar traumas.

Julie called Stella a true inspiration to her as a therapist.

TAKE-HOME POINTS

PTSD can be a debilitating disorder, and 8 percent of Americans (24.4 million) have PTSD at any given time.[30] The Veterans Stress Project, an initiative of the National Institute for Integrative Healthcare (NIIH), is determined to make a difference when it comes to PTSD related to combat or military service. They are a movement offering veterans free or low-cost sessions using EFT. To access the services, please visit www.stressproject.org. You can get in touch with a veteran who has used EFT to recover from PTSD through the website and read stories of their journey.

In a very exciting move, in October 2017 the U.S. Veterans Administration (VA) approved EFT. After reviewing the extensive evidence for the safety and efficacy of EFT, a group of experts in the VA's Integrative Health Coordinating Center published a statement approving EFT and several other complementary and integrative health (CIH) practices. They stated that based on the study by "the expert scientific community (both internal and external to VHA) knowledgeable about the safety of CIH approaches," EFT and several other methods including Healing Touch, acupressure, and Reiki, are "generally considered safe."[31]

EFT is remarkably quick to work and has the ability to efficiently pair a neutral or even calming response with a traumatic memory. This results in a unique detachment for the client, but one that gives them a great sense of control and ultimately peace. With a tool such as tapping available for returning war veterans, or in the hands of existing therapists, trauma may be more readily processed and complex syndromes might actually be avoided.

EFT, STRESS, AND ANXIETY

Technically speaking, stress is a physiological state: in a fight-or-flight situation, our bodies are ready to take on a threat or flee. (Modern research is suggesting this model of stress also includes the options of freeze or faint too). At some level, if we perceive an event or situation to be threatening, harmful, or something that will overtax our internal or external resources, then we tend to feel the sensations of stress.

You might be familiar with these physical sensations:

- Back pain
- Chest pain
- Heart palpitations
- Stomach upset
- Sleep problems
- Headaches

You may also have experienced such emotional states:

- Restlessness
- Worry

- Irritability

- Depression

- Sadness

- Anger

- Insecurity

- Lack of focus

- Burnout

- Forgetfulness

But what is stress? Pioneers in the area suggest stress is a process, a relationship between you and the environment.[1] We encounter a stressful event or situation, and we often ask ourselves, *What does it mean to me? Will I be okay?* The judgment we make tends to be one of the following:

- It's irrelevant (therefore I don't feel any stress)

- It's good (benign—I might even feel positive emotions)

- It's stressful (physical symptoms start)

Ultimately, we might be asking, *What kind of harm or loss might this situation cause me?* We actually keep reassessing the situation as time goes on (with the above questions) and decide on the same or a new decision based on the resources we have available for coping.

But when we have perceptions of uncertainty, feel a lack of control, and then engage in negative conversations in our head, this can lead to increased distress. The hormone most featured in the stress response is cortisol.

Cortisol, actually a steroid hormone, is produced from cholesterol in the two adrenal glands located on top of our kidneys. It is normally released in response to events and circumstances such as waking up in the morning, exercising, and also acute stress. It is best known for its role in the fight-or-flight response and is a survival mechanism that has stayed with us from our ancestors.

The problem is that cortisol is supposed to return to a normal level after a stressor is over. In today's world, however, a stressor may no longer be a threat from a wild animal. It might be not checking your phone or social media frequently, being overwhelmed by the loud person in the cubicle next to you at work every day, or finding the daily commute to and from work enough to make you want to quit your job. And the stressor might actually never end. This then leads to your body continually producing the stress hormone in case you need it to fight or flee.

Your body doesn't know that the reason you are stressed is the traffic jam; it just responds with the cortisol release. Too much cortisol leads to the body making extra glucose (that energy needed to fight or flee), which naturally increases blood sugar levels. It also reduces the body's inflammation response in those moments of stress (leading to sticky blood cells and plaque buildup), and lowered levels can affect the immune system over time. Long-term stress and elevated cortisol may also be linked to insomnia, chronic fatigue syndrome, thyroid disorders, dementia, and depression.

The long-term effect of stress can be toxic. And all you really wanted was the car in front of you to keep driving!

TYPES OF STRESS

What most people don't realize is that stress can actually be both positive (eustress) *and* negative (distress).

- *Eu*stress is deemed useful (e.g., your performance peaks with just the right amount of stress and cortisol). The relationship between arousal and performance was originally developed by psychologists Robert M. Yerkes and John Dillingham Dodson in 1908. They suggested that performance increases with physiological or mental arousal, but only up to a point. When levels of arousal become too high, performance decreases.

But simple tasks that don't tax us too much are not as affected.

- *Dis*tress is the term we often are referring to when we say we feel "stressed." It might be acute (short term) or chronic (long lasting). This is the one that results in the flood of hormones and potentially longer-term negative effects.

If stress is the result of the decision we make from that process above (and the reappraisal over time), anxiety, on the other hand, is a feeling of fear, worry, or unease. It may be a reaction to stress, or it can occur even if you can't identify a significant stressor.

Studies on EFT show that tapping can significantly lower the stress hormone cortisol after just one hour. It turns out it is highly effective to calm down the center in the brain that sends out the stress response, and the result can last longer over time than traditional therapies.

THE RESEARCH ON STRESS

A landmark study published in 2012 in the prestigious *Journal of Nervous and Mental Disease* found that EFT lowered cortisol significantly more than traditional talk therapy or resting.[2] The results showed that cortisol levels in the rest and therapy groups declined by an average of 14 percent, while the EFT group declined 24 percent. The decrease in cortisol was also associated with a corresponding decrease in psychological distress.

Thus the results indicated EFT had the ability to reduce the severity and range of psychological symptoms (particularly stress), and corresponding physiological reactions, in a sample of non-clinical participants. This was groundbreaking at the time.

In another study of 102 people from the general community who were attending a three-day EFT workshop, researchers found significant improvements in global and specific psychological distress (e.g., somatization, obsessive-compulsive, interpersonal sensitivity, depression, anxiety, hostility, phobic anxiety, para-noid ideation, psychoticism).[3] Everyone completed questionnaires about those symptoms one month before the workshop, imme-diately prior, immediately after the EFT workshop, and also one and six months later. At the six-month mark, global and specific improvements in psychological distress were maintained.

Based on the outcomes of this study, Dr. Dawson Church led a study that investigated 216 health-care workers who attended five professional conferences over a year.[4] They included alterna-tive-medicine practitioners, nonmedical personnel, chiropractors, and physicians (76 percent were female, and the average age was 48 years). The study was primarily measuring burnout in workers, and everyone received a two-hour workshop on EFT and then a two-hour session where they self-applied the technique.

Immediately before and after the workshop, participants com-pleted a measure of their pain levels, emotional distress, and food cravings. After the four hours, they reported significant improve-ments on all of these issues.

Everyone was contacted 90 days later to see if they had con-tinued to self-apply EFT once a week, three times a week, or not at all. What they found was that more use of EFT was associated with a steeper decrease in psychological symptoms, although not in symptom range or breadth. There were 70 people who indicated they were using EFT at least three times a week.

The results did support the previous study of community members and was found to be effective for issues typical in burn-out: pain, distress, and cravings. What was important about both these studies was that the people did not necessarily choose to attend an EFT intervention. They consented to the studies, but the roles of expectation and outcome may not have been present.

However, when people actively seek EFT treatment, the same type of outcomes occurs. Researchers in the United Kingdom con-ducted an evaluation of 39 individuals who sought out EFT treat-ment and attended an average number of five individual sessions in Sandwell.[5]

They also observed significant decreases in psychological distress, anxiety, and depression, in addition to improvement in well-being and self-esteem among the clients. What was also noteworthy was that only four to five sessions were required to observe an effect, possibly suggesting EFT to be a cost-effective treatment. This again supports the case that tapping works quickly and often more efficiently than comparable therapy approaches.

NOTES FROM A PRACTITIONER: STRESS

When Vivienne presented for therapy because of her overwhelming stress levels, she was very open to learning EFT. She had been a lawyer for over a decade and was on track to become a partner in her firm. However, this meant very long days; sometimes she slept at her desk, and the toll was visible. Her hair was falling out, she had a rash on her legs that was stress related according to the doctor, and she was emotionally eating fairly regularly.

To immediately start to calm her body, the therapist asked Vivienne to describe the stress symptoms she found hardest to cope with, and they started tapping with those. Examples included her constant pounding headache, feeling frustrated she couldn't easily fall asleep at night, and a general feeling of pressure on top of her shoulders.

This is an excellent way to start using EFT for stress. Start with the physical or emotional symptoms you can name, and tap to reduce their intensity. You might also know where it stems from, and including the sources in your setup phrases is advisable too.

Eventually Vivienne and her therapist started talking about her upbringing and messages in the family about working hard. They used tapping to process some of those memories as Vivienne realized her stress was a pattern in her life, and that by being stressed and overwhelmed, she actually earned the respect and admiration of her father.

The stress and workaholic pattern represented a tabletop (from Chapter 1), and the times in her life she recalled witnessing her father do the same were the legs to the table. There were also times (memories) where she did not achieve an outcome he expected, and the punishment was so severe that she decided when she was eight years old that she must always overachieve from that point forward to avoid the consequences. These were also other legs to the table, and the therapist helped her address those.

Over time the therapist and Vivienne were able to use tapping on the memories that still created distress for her, or where she had made a decision that no longer served her well. She was able to cut back her hours at work, her hair stopped falling out, and the rash disappeared. She decided against putting in her application to become a partner and instead started a new relationship. Work still fulfilled her, but she had more balance in her life; and funnily enough, her father didn't react negatively at all.

THE RESEARCH ON ANXIETY

An anxiety disorder is characterized by feelings of worry, anxiety, or fear to an extent that interferes in daily functioning, and it is one of the most common mental illnesses in America. It affects 18.1 percent of the population every year, and although it is highly treatable, only 36.9 percent of those suffering receive treatment.[6] We know sufferers are seeking help because people with an anxiety disorder are three to five times more likely to go to the doctor.

This is an area that has featured significantly in the EFT research studies. Because anxiousness is typically felt physically, tapping has become a useful strategy to calm the body.

One of the first large-scale studies involved 5,000 patients seeking treatment for anxiety across 11 clinics over a five-and-a-half-year period.[7] (This study was part of a larger investigation of more than 29,000 patients from 11 treatment centers in South America during a 14-year period.) Patients were allocated to a traditional psychological treatment, cognitive behavioral therapy (CBT) that included medication if needed, or acupoint treatment (precursor to TFT) with no medication.

Interviewers who were blind to the treatment modality placed each patient into one of three categories at the close of therapy, at 1 month, at 3 months, at 6 months, and at 12 months later. The three categories were no improvement with the presenting problem, some improvement, or complete remission. The raters did not know if the patient received CBT/medication or tapping. They only knew the initial diagnosis, the symptoms, and the severity, as judged by the intake assessment staff.

Complete remission was reported by 76 percent of the patients in the acupoint group and 51 percent of the CBT group (p < .0002). Some improvement to complete remission was reported by 90 percent of the patients in the acupoint group and 63 percent of the CBT group (p < .0002). Those 90 percent of acupoint patients improved *in an average of 3 sessions*, compared to an average of 15 sessions for the CBT patients. One year later 78 percent of the acupoint group maintained their improvements, compared with 69 percent of the CBT group.

Despite the large sample size and impressive outcomes, this study was initially an in-house assessment of a new method and was not designed with publication in mind. Not all the variables were controlled, and not all criteria were rigorously defined. Although record keeping was relatively informal, the study did use randomized samples, control groups, and double-blind assessment and is worthy of note because of the enormous differences between the approaches. For EFT to achieve the same outcomes as CBT in three sessions is incredible, and this study was really the start of these comparisons.

This study included an inspection of brain changes after treatment for anxiety. It was the first EFT study to do so and used pre- and post-treatment functional brain imaging (through computerized EEG, evoked potentials, and topographic mapping).[8] You can view the brain-scan images that were taken during four weeks of acupoint treatment for anxiety at innersource.net.[9]

A decrease in the intensity and frequency of generalized anxiety disorder (GAD) symptoms was associated with shifts toward normal levels of wave-frequency ratios in the brain's cortex. The pattern shown in the study's images was typical for GAD patients in the South American study who responded positively to the stimulation of acupoints.

The images in the study show the shift of red (highly dysfunctional waves) to blue (calmer state) in the central and frontal areas of the brain. This corresponded with a decrease in anxiety symptoms in intensity and frequency. Patients who received CBT with medication also showed similar changes in their scans, but they took a longer treatment time to achieve this.

What is also very important to note is that at one-year follow-up, the CBT patients' scans were more likely to have returned to their pretreatment levels than the acupoint patients. Furthermore, the patients who mainly only took antianxiety medication still reported a reduction of symptoms, but their brain scans did not show noticeable changes in the wave patterns. This may have indicated that the medication was suppressing the symptoms without addressing the underlying wave-frequency imbalances.

There have since been other tapping and anxiety studies, although many target these symptoms among other conditions, such as PTSD, as we saw in Chapter 4.

Headaches

In a group of 35 patients who were randomly allocated to either standard care (control group) or EFT for tension-type headaches, the EFT group reported significant reductions in perceived stress and the frequency and intensity of headaches.[10] They were instructed to use tapping twice a day for two months. The EFT patients also reported a significant improvement in their sleep after treatment.

The study did not have a long follow-up period (two months), and cortisol testing (saliva) did not show any differences between the two groups, but it was promising as a pilot.

Dental Patients

In a UK pilot investigation, 30 people awaiting dental treatment who had high anxiety (they scored 6+ on a scale of 0 to 10) received a brief 10-minute EFT session.[11] Dental-treatment anxiety affects between 10 and 30 percent of those seeking dental care, so it is a promising area for brief interventions. Patients indicated an average decrease of 5 points on the 0 to 10 scale, with 83 percent experiencing a decrease of at least 4 points. The study did not have a control group or a follow-up period, but at least indicated the same type of outcomes for brief EFT treatment as in other trials.

Another case series of four dental patients with high dental fear and one woman with anxiety about gagging (but low dental fear) received four weeks of EFT treatment (one hour each week).[12] All patients achieved normal scores on commonly feared dental stimuli at the end of the treatment; and at follow-up (seven and a half months later), they indicated the gains were held. The four high-dental-fear participants achieved reliable and clinically significant change on measures of trait dental fear and/or state dental anxiety, and, for three of them, on negative dental beliefs.

A 2017 pilot study also explored EFT as a treatment for dental anxiety.[13] Eight dental patients with anxiety were assigned to the EFT group or a nontreatment control condition (reading a golf magazine; four patients in each group). Each patient was asked to visualize being present in a dental chair while the researcher recounted aloud a list of dental triggers specific to each participant. They then completed anxiety assessments and engaged in a four-minute tapping intervention or read a magazine. After the four-minute intervention or reading period, they listened to the list of their specific dental triggers read aloud and were then retested while again listening to their list of triggers.

The average before and after anxiety scores of the control group differed by only three points (a decrease of 6 percent). However, the average anxiety scores for the EFT group decreased by 26 points (35 percent). While this was a very brief, one-session treatment, it indicated results similar to other trials and high-lighted the effectiveness of EFT to rapidly reduce dental anxiety.

Tapping may definitely be something to investigate for dental patients in the future. Although larger trials are needed to confirm the effectiveness, it appears promising. Again, very brief applications of EFT are needed to effect change; and in the cases where patients actively avoid attending a dentist even in the face of extreme pain or injury, successful ways to deal with this are needed.

Nursing Students

A pilot study of 39 nursing students enrolled in an associate degree nursing program was conducted in a two-year college in the southeastern region of the United States.[14] Those who volunteered learned EFT in a group setting and were encouraged to repeat it daily for stress and anxiety.

Self-reported anxiety was measured at baseline and then weekly for four weeks using the Perceived Stress Scale (PSS) and the State-Trait Anxiety Inventory (STAI). The students also completed a qualitative questionnaire at the end of the four weeks about their experiences. The STAI and PSS were administered weekly.

The researcher showed that EFT resulted in significant decreases in anxiety (p=.05), and the reduction in self-reported stress was statistically significant from the start to week four. The qualitative questionnaire also suggested that nursing students experienced a decrease in feelings of stress and anxiety, including a decrease in somatic symptoms.

Surgery Patients

Another study investigated the effectiveness of EFT for anxiety among women undergoing obstetric and gynecological surgeries.[15] Fifty women met the diagnostic criteria for moderate to severe anxiety; half were randomly allocated to the EFT group, and half to the control group. The modified Hamilton Anxiety Rating Scale was used to measure psychological and somatic anxiety.

The EFT group received two 10-minute EFT sessions. The first was on the day prior to surgery, and the second session was on the day of surgery. Both groups then received surgical treatment as usual.

The two groups were similar at the start with regards to anxiety, and immediately before surgery they were all reassessed. The control group did not have any change in anxiety; however, the anxiety scores in the EFT group decreased from 27.28 (± 2.47) to 7.60 (± 2.00) and were highly statistically significant ($p < 0.0001$). Their reductions in both psychological and somatic anxiety subscales were also significant ($p < 0.002$).

Given the high levels of stress and anxiety many people feel prior to surgery, EFT may be a cost-effective and brief intervention that has immense value in outcomes.

Public-Speaking Anxiety

In order to determine whether EFT was effective in reducing public speaking anxiety, 36 adults were randomly allocated to a treatment or wait-list group.[16] Given that this is such a common problem worldwide, studies like these are important. Everyone completed a Personal Report of Confidence as a Speaker (PRCS), a Personal Report of Communication Apprehension, the State-Trait Anxiety Inventory, a Timed Behavior Checklist, and their own SUD rating.

The wait-list participants attended a counseling service by appointment but did not receive any other intervention at first. The EFT intervention (delivered by one of three psychologists working in counseling and trained in EFT) was delivered over 45 minutes, and participants then delivered a four-minute speech in front of a small group. This was video recorded and later scored by independent observers blinded to treatment conditions on the Timed Behavior Checklist.

There were significant reductions for everyone in public-speaking anxiety on all the self-report measures but not on the behavioral observations. However, when the treatment group was examined alone, there were significant reductions in stated anxiety and the behavioral measures. Public-speaking confidence significantly increased in this group (p=0005), and there was a significant decrease (p=0.011) in general anxiety.

A significant reduction was also observed within the first 15 minutes of EFT, with further significant reductions also demonstrated at 30 and 45 minutes. EFT was found to be a quick and effective treatment for this type of anxiety.

Insomnia

It is well known that stressful life events are closely related to the occurrence of chronic insomnia. Greek researchers investigated stress and insomnia symptoms in 40 lawyers and allocated them to a stress-management technique program (which included progressive muscle relaxation, relaxation breathing technique, autogenic training, guided imagery, and EFT), or a wait-list (21 and 19 in the groups, respectively).[17]

The stress-management group experienced a statistically significant reduction in depression symptoms (p=0.015) and stress levels (p=0.029). They also reported moderate improvement in insomnia and sleep quality (effect sizes 0.3 and 0.32, respectively).

The Top Level: Meta-analysis

A meta-analysis of 14 randomized controlled trials of EFT for anxiety disorders investigated 658 people who had been treated with EFT or were in a control group.[18]

The researcher in charge found a very large treatment-effect size for EFT compared with the controls, who did not receive the treatment. It showed an effect size of d=1.23 (p < 0.001), while the effect size for combined controls was 0.41 (0.17–0.67, p=0.001). Even when accounting for the effect size of the control treatment, the EFT treatment was associated with a more significant decrease in anxiety scores.

What this means is that when d=1.23, 88 percent of the EFT treatment group was above the mean (average) of the control group. It also means 55 percent of the two groups overlapped, but that there was an 80 percent chance that a person picked at random from the treatment group would have a better score than a person picked at random from the control group. (For an illustration of what this looks like, please visit my website: www.peta stapleton.com.)

This was the first paper to report a meta-analysis of tapping for anxiety and clearly shows that EFT is a viable option for these conditions. It is not only cost effective because of the reduced sessions needed to achieve results, but it outperforms other approaches.

BEST PRACTICES FOR USING EFT WITH ANXIETY

In 2016 we surveyed a group of trained EFT practitioners to discover their experiences of working with clients with anxiety. The method we used is called a Delphi technique. This method involves using a group of participants or panelists who have particular expertise on a topic and consists of a series of at least two questionnaires or rounds of questions. The first round is used to generate ideas on a topic, from which a second-round questionnaire is developed. Additional rounds or questionnaires are used to further refine or reevaluate panelists' responses.

The whole idea is aimed at forming or exploring a consensus, whereby a certain number of panelists agree with each other on items. We used a consensus of at least 75 percent to indicate agreement.

We wanted to explore how skilled practitioners would define "best practice" for using EFT for anxiety in clients and the best EFT methods (or techniques) that should be used by EFT practitioners for anxiety in clients.

The practitioners shared that they believed the best practice for using EFT for anxiety issues should include the following:

- Building solid rapport with the client as a first step

- Being attuned to the client's body language, voice tone, and energy

- Completing a thorough assessment of anxiety symptoms

- Exploring with the client their current treatment for anxiety symptoms

- Exploring the client's family history

- Determining the client's own judgment of the severity of their anxiety symptoms (mild, moderate, etc.)

- Being mindful of the need to refer the client for help with more complex anxiety disorders (e.g., obsessive-compulsive disorder)

- As a practitioner, being competent in suicide prevention (complete extra training if needed)

- As a practitioner, having a thorough understanding of anxiety disorders (e.g., in the DSM-5) and their diagnostic criteria

Certain aspects were highlighted, such as teaching the client to tap on day-to-day triggers, including sights, sounds, smells, physical sensations, and thoughts. Tapping on any thoughts or feelings related to worries and anxieties about future situations was also recommended. If appropriate, engaging in tapping in combination with vivo exposure (in addition to imagined exposure) was recommended. This means a client would actually put themselves in a situation where the anxiety occurs (e.g., in an elevator if this was the fear) and do the tapping there. They would always advise to do this with a skilled practitioner for support.

They all agreed the best methods for using EFT for anxiety issues should include the following:

- Building solid rapport as a first step
- The "tell the story" technique, always paying attention to being very specific.
- Grounding techniques in addition to EFT (e.g., deep breathing, safe place visualization)
- The first and worst memory of anxiety
- Matrix Reimprinting technique (see Chapter 10)
- Daily tapping
- Continual tapping
- Engaging in EFT homework
- The "Gentle Techniques," such as including drawing in tapping processes (Many clients can feel their anxiety in a physical manner. They can be given a blank outline of a body and encouraged to draw on it where they feel their anxious sensations or feelings. They can then use these drawings to see how they progress with tapping.)
- Slow tapping (interestingly, fast tapping may feed into the anxiety loop, thus slowing it down can be useful)
- Checking the SUD rating regularly and teaching a client to do the same

NOTES FROM A PRACTITIONER: ANXIETY

John Freedom, chairman of the research committee for the Association for Comprehensive Energy Psychology, presents this case of working with a man with dental anxiety.[19]

"Michael" came to John with an unusual problem. He was experiencing a major fear of going to the dentist. Besides being a phobia, his anticipatory fear had become obsessive, in that it would attack him at odd times (not just when he had a dental appointment), and he could not get rid of it. Besides preventing him from going to the dentist (which he needed to do), it was also destroying his day-to-day peace of mind.

While this was clearly more than a simple phobia, treating the emotional aspects of the fear of dentists was the place to begin. John and Michael tapped a couple rounds on this fear of dentists. The intensity came down a few points [out of 10], but was still there.

John asked Michael, "Do you have a memory of dental pain or trauma that this fear is reminding you of?"

"Yes," Michael replied. He spoke of a memory that, as a young boy, he had chewed on some aluminum foil, causing an unpleasant pain.

They tapped several rounds on the aluminum-foil pain. It felt "lighter," but there was still more there. Michael mentioned having fear of a sudden pain, just coming out of nowhere. He said that he felt as though he had to keep his guard up at all times.

John asked Michael, "When you were a little boy, what used to happen to you that was sudden and unexpected?"

He thought for a moment, and then said, "My dad used to sometimes pick me up and just start spanking and hitting me, without warning." He reported feeling rather upset while telling this.

So John used these setup phrases:

- Even though Dad picked me up and spanked me unexpectedly . . .

- Even though I feel afraid of being attacked randomly and suddenly . . .

- Even though I've had to keep my guard up ever since . . .

- Even though I know that my dad is no longer alive, and that he wanted the best for me, in his own way, and I'm choosing to tap on myself, release these fears, and feel safe in my own body, now . . .

They then tapped on the spankings, on being picked up by Dad, and on this quality or aspect of being attacked suddenly and randomly.

"That feels much better!" Michael said after a few rounds of tapping. "But I don't know that it's totally gone. After all, I've had this issue for quite a while, and it just hits me out of the blue at random times."

John asked Michael, "If this random behavior were to have a positive purpose for you, what might that be?"

Michael replied, "Well, it has no positive purpose; it's a real drag."

John persisted, saying, "*If* it had a positive purpose for you, or a positive purpose for that young boy, what might that be?"

Michael thought a moment and said, "Well, I never really thought of it that way, but I've always felt like I've had to keep my guard up, and it may be trying to protect me in some odd way." He reported feeling an *aha!* and a shiver of recognition as he talked about this phobia trying to "protect" him.

Working on it from this angle, John guided him to say variations of the following:

- Even though I have this fear of being attacked suddenly and unexpectedly . . .

- Even though I've had to *keep my guard up* all the time . . .

- Even though I have to be very careful so someone doesn't attack me . . .

- Even though I know that my dad is no longer alive, and I'm okay now . . . I'm a strong, mature adult now, and no one is going to pick on me again . . . I survived! And even lived to tell the tale . . .

- And I'm choosing to forgive that little boy who believed he had to keep his guard up . . . to support and protect that little boy who's been so vigilant about protecting me ever since . . . to love and honor

and respect myself, for being so vigilant and so
watchful . . .

They did another few rounds of tapping, and Michael reported that not only was the fear of dentists and dental pain gone, but also that he now felt relieved because he understood why that fear was so obsessive. It was trying to warn him and protect him from danger. Recognizing that he was a strong adult now, and that it was unlikely that anyone would ever spank (or attack) him again, he realized that he could finally "let his guard down" and live in peace with himself.

Follow-up: John called Michael a few weeks later. He reported, "I think I'm doing really well; we really turned the corner on it. I can laugh about it now. It makes sense to me on an emotional level and hopefully on a deeper spiritual level . . ."

TAKE-HOME POINTS

Stress and anxiety can be debilitating to people who live with them every day. While a small amount of either can help you achieve and perform at your peak, it takes skill to control it and not let it run away (with you!). Experienced practitioners who work in this area are an untapped resource (no pun intended) when you want to know more about how to apply EFT to these issues.

While the latest research is showing it is how we *think* about stress and worry that determines whether it has a negative effect on us, the addition of EFT for these symptoms may go a long way to helping sufferers achieve that state of calm.[20]

EFT AND DEPRESSION

The World Health Organization suggests major depressive disorder, or depression, is the fourth leading cause of disability worldwide. There are an estimated 350 million people of all ages suffering, and approximately 16.2 percent of the world's adult population experiences at least one depressive episode during their lifetime.[1]

Anyone who has felt the depths of these dark episodes will know that they might do anything to relieve the feeling. My colleagues and I often hear statements like this from patients about their concerns:

> *I have been doing some Google research into some issues I face and have learned it could be depression. I have also discovered my mother's postnatal depression and lack of realizing it till I was eight could be a factor in this. I noticed the study you're doing, and I am in desperate need to know if my beliefs are substantiated or if I am in fact just trying to find someone to blame that isn't me. I hope to hear back from you, as it is a very complicated situation—well, it seems it is, and I am struggling to know where to turn.*

. . . .

I am interested in assisting with the program for adults suffering depression . . . I have been diagnosed by my GP a few years ago as suffering from depression and anxiety. I am single, never married or had children, and try to endure natural endorphins to assist with my systems (e.g., bike riding, try to laugh at silly life things). I do not sleep well; average data says you should sleep six to eight hours for an adult. I am interested in this eight-week treatment program at Bond University.

My name is _____ and I'm 23 years old. I feel like I'm always upset, depressed, or angry; and I don't know what to do to get out of this cycle. My partner advised me to see a psychologist, and that's how I came across your website. I read about the technique you will use to treat depression, and I would like to be a part of it.

The following signs and symptoms are considered indicators of depression if they persist for a period of more than two weeks:

- Feeling sad or empty most of the day, nearly every day
- Reduced interest and pleasure in activities and perhaps withdrawal from friends and activities once enjoyed
- Increased irritability or agitation
- Significant unintentional weight loss or gain or a change in appetite
- Oversleeping or undersleeping, lack of enthusiasm, low energy or motivation
- Missed school or poor school performance
- Poor self-esteem or feeling inappropriately guilty
- Feeling worthless or hopeless
- Recurrent thoughts of death or suicide

STUDIES OF SYMPTOMS

Depression is an emerging area in EFT research, as it represents a complex clinical concern. Some studies previously mentioned in other chapters highlight that depressive symptoms remit after other conditions are treated too. We discuss some of the studies here, but those more relevant to PTSD or other conditions feature in those particular chapters. Let's start with students.

Depression in American College Students

In 2012, American researchers assessed 238 first-year college students using the Beck Depression Inventory and found 30 students met the criteria for moderate to severe depression.[2] They were randomly assigned to either an EFT treatment or control group. The EFT group received four 90-minute group sessions of tapping, whereas the control group received nothing.

Those who received EFT were found to have significantly less depression three weeks later, with an average depression score in the nondepressed range following treatment, compared to the control group who demonstrated *no change* in depressive symptoms. Cohen's d was 2.28, indicating an *extremely strong* effect size.

Note that this study was limited in that it didn't have an active comparison treatment group, and the follow-up period wasn't very long, but it did highlight the potential usefulness of EFT as a therapy for depression.

Australian Adults with Major Depressive Disorder

Some of my own research included an initial study of EFT to treat major depressive disorder in adults in a group setting. My team and I wanted to know exactly what needed to be included in an EFT program to achieve outcomes.[3]

In this study the Mini-International Neuropsychiatric Interview (MINI) was used to diagnose psychiatric disorders in participants. This is administered by a psychologist. They also completed the Beck Depression Inventory-II, Depression Anxiety Stress Scales, and demographic information. Eleven adults were recruited and needed to have a diagnosis or probable diagnosis of major depressive disorder. We confirmed the diagnosis with the MINI; however, only 10 of the 11 adults met criteria.

The additional participant did not meet diagnostic criteria for either major depressive disorder or an alternate disorder, but was accepted into the treatment group due to self-reported depressive symptoms. At the time we felt it was the ethical thing to do.

The 11 adults then attended an eight-week, 16-hour group treatment program. This was two hours per week. Just a note here: If a participant in our trials was taking medication for depression (or anything else), they kept taking it for our treatment program. We do not ever suggest they change this without consulting their medical practitioner or specialist. All participants were also given contact details for counseling support services and suicide hotlines to access outside of weekly sessions.

The first hypothesis asked whether Clinical EFT resolved major depressive disorder as a diagnosis. The data revealed that while the diagnosis was not completely resolved immediately after eight weeks for everyone, two members no longer met criteria. In addition, all 11 adults no longer met diagnosis for *one or more other disorders* they had when they started. These were disorders such as social anxiety disorder, obsessive-compulsive disorder, and generalized anxiety disorder. So EFT impacted those diagnoses through our program too.

The second hypothesis asked whether Clinical EFT was effective at reducing the symptoms of major depressive disorder. In several cases individual adults reported clinical differences in symptoms. That is, the difference was enough so that if measured in a clinical setting, it would indicate treatment was successful. Therefore a clinically valid difference was achieved.

The third hypothesis asked whether the treatment effects of Clinical EFT were sustained after three months. Improvements *were* maintained, and many of the group members experienced a continual improvement in their symptoms over time.

Group members were also asked about their experience of the program each week. This survey indicated 88 percent found the Clinical EFT program information and skills to be useful, and 100 percent found the information easy to understand and apply. This was a starting point, as this trial was only a pilot and did not have a comparison or control group. However, the nature of EFT to affect other comorbid conditions or co-occurring symptoms became evident.

COMPARING EFT TO A GOLD STANDARD FOR TREATMENT OF DEPRESSION

At the completion of that study, we compared EFT to CBT (a gold standard therapy) for sufferers of depression. Ten adults from the community were randomly assigned to an eight-week, 16-hour CBT or EFT group program, and all screened positive for a primary diagnosis of major depressive disorder using the MINI.[4] We also included 57 members from the community who did not have any diagnosis, to see if the treatments would compare to their [normal] scores on measures of depression.

The eight sessions for both treatment programs were structured as follows:

- Session 1: Psychoeducation regarding the treatment approach

- Session 2: Behaviors involved in the maintenance of depression

- Session 3: The thinking-feeling connection

- Session 4: Cognitive restructuring (changing the way you think)

- Session 5: Core beliefs (which often come from childhood years)

- Session 6: Stress and relaxation training

- Session 7: Goal setting

- Session 8: Self-management (relapse prevention)

Two of the four participants in the CBT group and three of the six participants in the EFT group no longer met the diagnostic criteria for major depression at the end of the eight weeks. So effectively they both achieved results for 50 percent of each group. However, findings showed that the CBT group reported a significant reduction in depressive symptoms at the end of the eight weeks, but this *was not maintained over time.*

The EFT group reported a delayed effect and indicated a significant reduction in depression symptoms at the three- and six-month follow-up points. They did not report any differences over the eight weeks, but symptom reduction seemed to happen afterward. After six months, they were *still* reporting an absence of symptoms.

While this study was small and the first to examine and compare the effectiveness of a gold standard approach and EFT in reducing depression among adults, the findings did indicate that EFT may be an effective treatment strategy worthy of further investigation.

ADDRESSING OTHER ISSUES AFFECTS DEPRESSION LEVELS

Weight loss: As mentioned, depression symptoms can also improve when EFT is applied for other symptoms. This highlights the interplay of different conditions, and perhaps the overlap that occurs. Research has shown a link between levels of the stress hormone cortisol and both depression and obesity. Elevated cortisol levels are linked to centrally distributed adipose tissue, and depression is also associated with elevated cortisol.[5,6]

In one of our food-craving/weight-loss studies, we found depressive symptoms improved with weight loss.[7] There were 96 adults who underwent a four-week, eight-hour EFT treatment for their food cravings, and all were overweight or obese. This study is described more in the chapter on food and weight issues, but what we found was the significant improvements in depressive and obsessive symptoms, interpersonal sensitivity (ability to accurately assess others' abilities, states, and traits from nonverbal cues), psychoticism (a personality pattern typified by aggressiveness), and hostility that occurred during the four weeks were maintained 12 months later. As food cravings improved, so did all these other symptoms.

What this study highlighted was the potential role mental-health conditions might play in successful maintenance of weight loss, particularly the link between depression and weight loss.

Health-care workers: As mentioned in Chapter 5, EFT also impacted the psychological distress levels, pain, and cravings in 218 health-care workers who self-applied tapping for two hours.

Emotional conditions: UK researchers have also found EFT to reduce anxiety, depression, anger, and other emotions in a review of people seeking therapy (see Chapter 5).

THE META-ANALYSIS

A meta-analysis has also occurred for EFT and depression. It examined 20 studies and included outcome studies (with 446 people), as well as randomized clinical trials (a total of 653 people: 306 EFT and 347 control subjects).[8]

EFT demonstrated a very large effect size (Cohen's d across all studies was 1.31) in the treatment of depression. At the end of EFT treatment, Cohen's d for the randomized trials was 1.85 and for outcome studies was 0.70.

Effect sizes for follow-ups less than 90 days was 1.21, and for greater than 90 days it was 1.11. These both indicate very large sizes.

This meant 90 percent of the treatment group was above the mean (average) of the control group, and there was an 82 percent chance that a person picked at random from the treatment group would have a better score than a person picked at random from the control group. The average amount of depression symptom reductions across all studies was 41 percent.

EFT was also more effective than diaphragmatic breathing, as well as psychological interventions such as supportive interviews and sleep-hygiene education. EFT was also superior to treatment as usual and achieved results in time frames ranging from 1 to 10 sessions. No significant treatment effect difference between EFT and EMDR was found (they achieved similar outcomes). Given what I discussed about Van der Kolk's stance on somatic therapies for PTSD, including EMDR and EFT, it is not unusual to see these achieving similar results.

What is interesting is that the effect size for EFT (d=1.31) was larger than that measured in meta-analyses of antidepressant drug trials and psychotherapy studies.

EFT produced very large treatment effects for depression whether delivered in a group or individual format, and participants maintained their gains over time. This is very hard to ignore since the results are there. Including EFT in the treatment of depression should be essential.

BEST PRACTICES FOR USING EFT WITH DEPRESSION

In 2016 we surveyed a group of trained EFT practitioners to look at their experiences of working with clients with depression (the Delphi study). This was the same study highlighted at the end of Chapter 5, as this group of skilled professionals responded about anxiety and depression as two separate conditions in clients. We explored how these skilled practitioners defined "best practice" for using EFT for depression in clients, and the best EFT methods (or techniques) they recommended should be used by EFT practitioners for depression in clients. The outcomes are shared here.

Ideas for Working with Depression: First Steps

- Build solid rapport with the client as a first step. We noticed depressed adults were difficult to keep engaged throughout our eight-week group program too. If their energy was low, they wanted to stay home and not attend (despite wanting to overcome their depression). We used daily short messages (texts) in between sessions to stay in touch with them and remind them to attend the next session. If they didn't, we immediately followed up with a telephone call.

- Do a thorough assessment of depression symptoms in the beginning, using valid measures if you can.

- Have training in suicide prevention and self-harm in case this is an issue for the client (provide details of crisis services for support in between sessions if needed, and complete safety plans too).

- Explore the person's current treatment for depression and if medicated, do not make any changes without consultation from a medical/specialist practitioner.

- Explore family history and whether diagnosis or treatment has occurred for other members.

- Determine the client's judgment of the severity of their depression symptoms (mild, moderate, severe).

- Have a willingness to refer to another health professional if needed.

- Connect with client's general practitioner or specialist (e.g., psychiatrist) as a standard process to let them know of your own treatment plans (e.g., written letter).

Ideas for Working with Depression: Treatment Issues

- Grounding techniques are highly recommended
  in the beginning before using tapping. This might
  be things like breathing only, progressive muscular
  relaxation, using the five senses to ground oneself, or
  even mindfulness-based approaches.

- Use body/physical sensations as basis for tapping in
  the beginning. This might be using a setup statement
  such as "Even though I feel exhausted and my body
  aches, I accept myself anyway."

- Use slow tapping with clients, as it will match their
  energy state to begin with. It may become faster
  over time.

- Suggest clients do tapping daily, on anything to begin
  with. This will make it more habitual.

- Use "gentle and tearless" techniques in tapping (see
  www.eftuniverse for more detail on these styles),
  which will allow clients to slowly sneak in on their
  issues and potential precipitating events. Gentle
  techniques allow the process to go at the client's own
  pace and help with regulating intense distress.

- Consider 9 Gamut, a process in the original
  version of EFT. This involves eye movements and is
  recommended for intense depression and symptoms.

- Consider dividing the client's sessions into two per
  week. This may help them preserve their energy and
  allow some space in between for consolidation of any
  shifts they make.

- Investigate secondary-benefit issues that might be
  present. These are reasons to not change or stay the
  same. We often phrase it, "What is the upside to
  staying this way?"

- Give clients videos (perhaps of the practitioner) of tapping to watch in between sessions, in case they cannot remember the process due to the nature of depression affecting their memory. Just watching someone else tap on a video results in the client's mirror neurons firing, and they may still receive a benefit.

- Finally, follow solid protocols for using EFT for depression. Look at what the research says works, and if in doubt, seek supervision or mentoring.

NOTES FROM A PRACTITIONER

Roy was a 55-year-old man who presented to me specifically to learn more about tapping for his depression. He had a long history of clinical depression, including many hospitalizations and inpatient treatment. But nothing had really worked. He had previously learned a little bit about tapping through Internet searches but felt at a loss to engage in using it on his own. The first session outlined the technique and also took a full history of Roy's story.

Roy's recollection was that he had been depressed most of his adult life, and perhaps even in his adolescence. It had taken its toll on his marriage, and his wife was ready to leave. He reported he had a successful health business for many decades, teaching others in the coaching and lifestyle area, but recently it too had declined.

Some basic tapping on how Roy felt about his depression (e.g., angry at being depressed for so long) resulted in him questioning *why* he was so depressed. He used this statement in the tapping setup and focused on "why am I so depressed." His statement was "Even though I don't know why I am so depressed, I accept myself anyway." This resulted in an angry feeling and this was added to the setup statement.

As he focused on the angry feeling and the questioning of "why," Roy remembered something from his childhood. This surprised him, as he was not thinking of this at the time.

He recalled that when he was eight years old, the family moved from a colder rural area to a warmer climate a long distance away, because his younger brother had asthma. He recalled the doctor had recommended the move because the damp environment in the country was not helping his brother, while a warmer climate might help. So his parents made this decision.

Several things stood out for Roy when he remembered this:

- He became aware that his depressed feelings started shortly after they moved. He felt this was the beginning of these symptoms, not later in adolescence.

- He recalled feeling angry and powerless. He didn't want to move away from his friends at school, and he was furious his parents did not talk with all of the family members about the decision.

- He actually felt angry toward his younger brother, although he knew it wasn't his fault. He buried the resentment and angry feelings toward his brother for having asthma deep inside.

- He realized why he had distanced himself from his family since leaving home. He may have been unconsciously punishing them for the move and his brother's asthma.

All of these issues were targeted with tapping, and Roy was able to release these long-held distressing feelings as they came to the surface. Over the next year, Roy was able to begin to feel some positive emotions for the first time since he was eight years old, and he questioned whether he actually felt depressed anymore.

His wife supported him through the process, and his adult children visited often as they said they enjoyed his company more than ever. Business picked up, and Roy started to feel like life was worth living again and living fully. He no longer had days in bed; and after 18 months, he felt compelled to reach out to his younger brother, and they reconnected as adults.

TAKE-HOME POINTS

In my experience, the treatment of depression in adults is multifaceted. Some need to do tapping on regaining interest or pleasure in activities; others target sleep issues and energy levels. While global tapping scripts can be a good starting point, being very specific about what contributes to a person's individual situation is vital.

EFT, FOOD CRAVINGS, AND WEIGHT ISSUES

Food cravings and weight issues are where all my EFT research started, and much of the research you will read here is mine. Not because there isn't any other research, it's just that I have conducted many trials in this area. Since embarking on investigating the usefulness of tapping for food and weight issues, I often receive these types of e-mails:

> *I saw with interest the results of your recent diet trial on Channel 9 this evening. I go to the gym four to five times a week, do weights, pump class, boxing, and kick boarding. I eat healthily and only drink occasionally. But—and the big but—is my sweet tooth: lollies, chocolate. My BMI [body mass index] is approximately 28, and I am seven to eight kilos over my ideal weight. I am fit but fat.*

. . . .

> *I am interested in taking part in the trial. My BMI is 44. I have been overweight most of my life; and on two occasions,*

I have managed to lose 60 kilos, and then put it back on both times. I am constantly craving food (especially sweets), and I hope your program can help me. Apart from my weight, I am in great health. I hope to hear from you soon.

Research tells us that if you get a food craving, you will probably end up eating that food. Food cravings are also associated with higher weight and a stronger preference for high-fat food.

The obesity crisis in Australia has become worse in the last decade: 63.4 percent of Australian adults are overweight or obese, and this is well over half of the nation's population.[1] That's almost two in three adults. One report found that Australia is one of the most obese nations in the world, with one in four Australian children ranking as overweight or obese too.[2]

Across the globe, obesity has more than doubled since 1980. The World Health Organization says 39 percent of adults aged 18 years and over were overweight in 2014, and 13 percent were obese. Most of the world's population lives in countries where being overweight and obese kills more people than being underweight. What is worst is that 41 million children under the age of five were overweight or obese in 2014.[3]

You can see why I wanted to investigate the effectiveness of EFT for weight loss!

OUR FIRST AUSTRALIAN RESEARCH TRIAL

When I first decided to offer EFT treatment for food cravings in overweight and obese adults through a research trial, my then-superior said no one would attend.

After I appeared on a national current-affairs show to "advertise" the study (which was free), we had over 4,500 people call, e-mail, or write to be included. This was after I demonstrated the strange act of tapping for a chocolate muffin, so they knew what they were in for.

My boss never said another word, of course.

We ended up with 96 overweight and obese adults with severe food cravings and randomized them into either a four-week, eight-hour EFT treatment program or a wait-list (where they did receive the EFT treatment but only after the other group finished).[4] As I've mentioned, a wait-list allows us to see whether time affects any symptoms (e.g., maybe food cravings would go away with time). They didn't.

We measured everyone's weight and body mass index, the degree of food cravings, each individual's perception of the power of food over them, and their restraint capabilities and psychological symptoms at the start, end, 6 months later, and 12 months later. While we weighed everyone at the beginning and end of the trial, we relied on self-report for the follow-up periods.

Every factor we measured significantly improved. The average weight loss over the 12 months was statistically significant (approximately 5.05 kilograms, or 11.1 pounds). It was in this study that we also saw those improvements mentioned in the previous chapter in depressive and obsessive symptoms, interpersonal sensitivity, psychoticism, and hostility, which were all maintained 12 months following treatment.

We started to hear things like this:

Amazingly I haven't had a bar of chocolate in two weeks, since I tapped on it!! Coke Zero and salt-and-vinegar chips have gone too, after many, many years of relying on them!

. . . .

I found the program extremely enlightening, and it has helped me with some deep-seated emotional issues that I have carried since childhood (some 70 years).

In the same study, a small group of the EFT people (40) were compared to 7 people who were randomly allocated to cognitive behavioral therapy (CBT), a psychoeducation intervention (7), or a wait-list group (40). This was a preliminary study to assess the effectiveness of EFT against CBT, the gold standard psychological treatment. The results indicated that the CBT group resulted in a significant reduction in total food cravings after the four-week treatment and an increase in the participants' power over food. An increase in restraint ability after treatment also occurred for the psychoeducation group.

But the EFT group indicated significant reductions on *all measures after treatment*, except restraint ability. Increased restraint was significant, however, at the 6- and 12-month points, indicating a time lag.

Because of these outcomes, we then embarked on a larger trial that compared EFT to CBT. We were beginning to consider the idea that perhaps tapping was going to be at least comparable to a gold standard treatment in this area, if not superior.

EFT AGAINST A GOLD STANDARD

In 2014 my team and I began another trial. There were 83 overweight or obese adults who were randomly allocated to an eight-week EFT or CBT intervention.[5] This was important, as it meant there was an absence of bias: no one was able to choose the treatment they received.

As you can imagine, chocolate was the most commonly craved food by the group (53 percent), followed by sweet carbohydrates (e.g., cakes, cookies, soft drinks; 15.7 percent), other carbohydrates (neither sweet nor salty, like bread; 15.7 percent), salty foods (e.g., chips, salted nuts; 14.5 percent), and caffeinated items such as coffee (1.2 percent). The majority of adults said they experienced cravings on a daily basis (83.1 percent), with 67.5 percent indicating that they would consume their craving every day.

The Setup of the Trial

Our team weighed all participants in the first session of their group and had them complete questionnaires relating to the severity of their food craving, each individual's perception of the power of food over them, their restraint capabilities, and psychological symptoms such as anxiety and depression.

The treatment was then offered in two-hour sessions once per week in small groups of 10 to 15 participants (EFT or CBT). A control community group of 92 normal-weight adults was utilized for comparison to see if the two treatment groups could reach normalized scores on the outcome measures above.

Here is an overview of what we typically do in these sessions:

- Session 1 described the type of treatment participants were to receive (EFT or CBT) and gave examples of how it would be applied.

- Session 2 discussed the nature of food cravings and how they happen. Cravings are described as an *emotional and physiological intense urge* (to eat). This session introduced the fact that mental imagery may be a key component of food cravings (i.e., when people crave a specific food, they have vivid images of that food in their mind).

- Session 3 outlined the nine primary emotions (i.e., anger, sadness, surprise, fear, distress, disgust, guilt, shame, and interest) and their relationship to emotional eating and cravings.

- Session 4 taught about limiting beliefs (irrational versus rational thinking) and how to change them in relationship to emotional eating and cravings. The EFT group used the tapping sequence when they recognized a negative thought, while the CBT group was taught to substitute a more useful thought for the negative one.

- Session 5 described the differences between distress versus eustress, and how these concepts impact emotional eating and cravings. The EFT group tapped on the feelings of stress and how they felt about this to achieve a calmer physical state, while the CBT group were taught muscular relaxation and deep breathing.

- Session 6 focused on goal setting and summarized how limiting beliefs can impact goal achievement (especially related to weight loss). The EFT group engaged in the tapping process for any limiting beliefs they noticed when they set a goal, while the CBT group was taught the SMART goal-setting formula and taught to substitute neutral or more positive thoughts for negative or unhelpful ones.

  SMART is an acronym representing these words:
  S: specific
  M: measurable, meaningful, motivational
  A: agreed upon, attainable, achievable, action-oriented
  R: realistic, relevant, reasonable, rewarding, results-oriented
  T: time-based, timely, tangible.

- Session 7 discussed concepts around good nutrition and the establishment of regular eating. Both groups were given the same information, but the EFT group engaged in tapping around any feelings they had about eating a healthier diet (e.g., deprivation), while the CBT group was taught to recognize their thoughts and feelings and substitute more helpful and appropriate ones.

- Session 8 discussed common and specific triggers and warning signs that might indicate a relapse was imminent, and how to manage these in the future. Both groups identified their own individual triggers for food cravings, and all skills were reviewed with the view to still use them posttreatment.

At the end of eight weeks, we again measured everyone's weight (converted to body mass index too), the severity of food cravings, each individual's perception of the power of food over them, their restraint capabilities, and psychological symptoms (such as anxiety and depression).

What Happened?

Overall, EFT and CBT demonstrated *comparable effectiveness* in reducing food cravings, one's responsiveness to food in the environment (power of food), and dietary restraint, with Cohen's effect size values suggesting moderate-to-high practical significance for both interventions. These gains were also maintained 6 and 12 months following the interventions.

This was quite an achievement, as it showed EFT could be *as effective as a gold standard approach*. The research community likes to see these studies as a starting point.

Both the EFT and CBT treatments were capable of producing reductions in food cravings, the power of food, and dietary restraint that matched *the scores of a nonclinical community sample.* These were adults who were normal weight without any cravings.

Psychological Outcomes

In the same study, we also examined psychological factors using the Patient Health Questionnaire.[6] This particular questionnaire has five modules covering five common types of mental disorders, including depression, anxiety, somatoform, alcohol, and eating modules. We were very interested in the amount of anxiety, depression, and somatic symptoms (anything physically felt in the body) our participants were experiencing.

- *Anxiety:* The CBT group had significantly lower anxiety scores at the end of the eight-week group program, but this effect was not maintained at 6- and

12-month follow-up points. It was not significantly different at those time points than levels before CBT.

However, the EFT group reported a significant decrease in anxiety and this reduction was maintained at 6- and 12-month follow-ups. Effectively the EFT intervention was better at impacting the anxiety symptoms than the CBT treatment.

- *Depression:* While the CBT group participants had significantly higher depressive symptoms prior to starting their treatment, they did not report any significant decreases in their depression scores from pre-intervention to any follow-up measurement point. The EFT group, however, reported significant decreases in their depression symptoms over the eight weeks and all follow-up points.

- *Somatic symptoms:* The CBT participants had significantly higher somatic symptoms at the start of their treatment and reported significantly decreased somatic scores across the eight weeks, and this was maintained at 6- and 12-month follow-up points. The EFT group did not report any significant decreases in symptoms at all. This may have been a function of having lower symptoms to begin with, which affects whether any change occurs.

Overall, the results of this aspect of the study revealed that EFT was indeed capable of producing reductions in anxiety and depression symptoms, and was not only comparable to gold standard approaches such as CBT, but superior in some aspects. It also showed that psychological intervention is beneficial for treating comorbidities in obesity and points to the role mental-health issues may play in this area.

WHAT WE LEARNED FROM EXAMINING FOOD DIARIES

In our early four-week trial, we looked at food diaries from 89 female overweight and obese adults.[7] Those diaries indicated that the most common reasons women suggested they were eating included wastage, emotion, and reward.

Wastage applied to any reason for eating relating to discarding food. Examples included "I couldn't waste it," and "There were leftovers."

Reward was indicated through responses such as "I didn't have a chocolate this morning," and "Just got home from work, so I deserved it."

Any emotion which appeared to trigger the food to be eaten was coded as an emotive reason. Examples included "bored" and "felt bad."

Across both the 7- and 14-day analyses, the majority of cravings were occurring between one and three times per day, and more than 50 percent of participants indicated SUD ratings higher than 5 out of 10 across a 7-day period, and 40 percent higher than a 5 across a 12-day period. These women were clearly struggling with frequency and intensity of cravings.

Addressing Wastage

Eating food because of wastage was actually *the strongest* reason cited and was of particular interest given the majority of women in the study were aged 41 to 56-plus years.

We noted anecdotally while conducting the treatment groups that these women had great difficulty discarding food once they had dealt with the craving issue through the EFT procedure. Even though they openly reported they did not want to eat the craved food anymore as it had lost its appeal through tapping, they most definitely did *not* want to throw the food out. What emerged were the long-held beliefs and emotions about "wasting food," which they had mostly learned from their mothers and grandmothers. Historically, these predecessors were women who grew up in the

Great Depression era of the 1930s and World Wars I and II, where food may have been scarce. Famine was very common, and to waste food would have been unheard of.

The waste theme in the studied food diaries confirmed these observations. Diary entries, which highlighted these themes, included the following:

> *Daughter and I made scones to eat because there's cream in fridge. Great to cook with her, but thinking I should have just thrown the cream out rather than make and buy things to have with it (bought strawberries too). Realized definitely having cream in house makes it so I can't think of having any other food, but I just can't throw food out.*

. . . .

> *Babysat grandchild, and she ate lollies. I had three. Feeling like a naughty child. She wanted some cake at café, and I ate the leftovers.*

The field of epigenetics, which means "above genetics," is now suggesting that the effects of a grandparent's lifestyle or diet could have been passed down, not through their genes, but through something beyond their genes. The effects of maternal nutrition or other environmental "exposures" are well recognized; therefore in the nutritional field, epigenetics is exceptionally important, because food intake can modify epigenetic phenomena and alter the expression of genes.

Based on this knowledge, it was no surprise that the women in the treatment groups had ingrained reactions toward going without food, wasting food, and even hoarding it "just in case." This may have been very relevant to their ancestors, but not so much in the current food-abundant lifestyle of today.

First, environments that are nutritionally limited (e.g., during the Great Depression in the 1930s) may mismatch individuals later in life when food-dense environments are now available. A woman pregnant after the two world wars, who may have grown up in a time of famine and then exposed her child to an early life of food scarcity, may have altered epigenetic mechanisms involved in the obesity susceptibility in the child.

A second possible pathway is that of fetal or infant overnutrition resulting in adult obesity (e.g., a woman who lived through World War II and had a child after the war, then compensated for her own undernutrition by overfeeding her child). That child would now be over 50 years of age and living in a very energy-dense environment. And those children were the women in our trials.

Our study of these food diaries in overweight and obese adults highlighted the importance of addressing the issue of *food wastage and the feelings associated with it*, as well as eating in response to emotion or as a reward in weight-loss treatment programs.

This became a very important feature to address.

THE MOVE TO ONLINE TRIALS

After we established EFT for food issues in overweight/obese adults was comparable to a gold standard and lasted at least for the next 12 months, we decided to test its effectiveness in an online format.[8] We envisaged being able to reach people in rural and remote areas.

Web-based technologies offer enormous potential for increasing community members' access to evidence-based health and well-being services, as well as offering therapists increased choice and flexibility in delivering services to populations where previous access has been poor.

Therefore we conducted a worldwide study of 314 adults (96.17 percent females, 3.83 percent males) who engaged in an EFT treatment online, and a wait-list control group of 254 adults who waited for treatment to see if the impact of time affected their food cravings. (It didn't.)

Participants completed an eight-week online EFT intervention targeting food cravings, dietary restraint, the subjective power of food, weight, somatic symptom severity, anxiety, and depression symptoms.

For the EFT group, sweet carbohydrates (e.g., cakes, cookies, soft drinks) were the most commonly craved foods (33.8 percent), followed by carbohydrates that are neither sweet nor salty (e.g., bread; 18 percent), chocolate (15.7 percent), salty foods (e.g., chips, salted nuts; 12.8 percent), and caffeinated items (2 percent). Two-thirds of these participants reported that they experienced cravings on a daily basis (65.9 percent), and 49.2 percent consumed their craving on a daily basis.

The group that was waiting for treatment revealed sweet carbohydrates were the most commonly craved foods as well (32 percent), followed by salty foods (18.9 percent), carbohydrates that are neither sweet nor salty (17.1 percent), chocolate (13.2 percent), and caffeinated items (1.3 percent). The majority reported that they experienced cravings on a daily basis (70.6 percent), with 48.2 percent saying they would consume their stated craving on a daily basis.

The Setup of the Online EFT Program

The EFT treatment intervention consisted of 32 video lessons across seven modules that were professionally recorded and featured myself as the therapist. Each module comprised three to eight lessons, and participants were instructed to limit themselves to one lesson per day and no more than one module per week in order to more fully engage in each topic; to avoid burnout; to maintain motivation throughout the entire course; and to make better neurological, psychological, and physical adaptations over time.

Participants were able to repeat the lessons as many times as they wanted and review past videos at any stage in the course. The length of the recorded lessons varied between approximately 2 and 15 minutes, and participants were required to complete a lesson quiz before progressing to the next video in each module. This ensured all videos were viewed and participants did not avoid any.

The topics of the weekly modules were (1) introduction to EFT, (2) tapping on less healthy foods, (3) tapping on healthier foods, (4) tapping on emotional eating, (5) tapping on increasing the desire for physical activity, (6) tapping on drinks, and (7) tapping into mindful-intuitive eating.

The first video of each module consisted of an introduction to that week's topic. The specific strategy involved participants focusing on their craving and associated emotions and using the tapping method during the treatment. If they were tapping on food or drink in that module, they were asked to have it in front of them (exposure) and to do the video at the time of day they usually consumed it. This was important for alcoholic drinks, for example.

Participants were also encouraged to use EFT outside of watching the recorded lessons during times of craving, if they required it.

What Happened?

We found significant reductions on *all of the questionnaire measures* for participants in the EFT condition, with no significant differences for participants in the wait-list control group. After the wait-list also completed the program, we collapsed the groups together to analyze the data as a whole group. Follow-up analyses at 6 and 12 months revealed significant reductions across the eight weeks *on all measures*. Every single aspect we measured changed significantly and stayed changed a year later.

Analyses also revealed that as individuals' food cravings improved, *their symptoms of anxiety and depression improved*. This mirrored what we had found in the in-person trial with psychological symptoms and food cravings.

This study was the first clinically researched trial of online delivery of EFT for weight management and provided preliminary findings of the utility of online EFT as an adjunct tool in the fight against obesity worldwide. It meant that offering EFT in online spaces does result in significant change for people, and as long as the program being delivered is specific, focused, and based on a sound understanding of the topic being presented, it will work.

ONLINE DELIVERY COMPARED TO IN-PERSON EFT

After conducting EFT trials both in-person and one online, we were interested in whether there was a difference in style of delivery in achieving outcomes for participants. Therefore we compared the two separate randomized controlled trials, because each program utilized the same Clinical EFT intervention targeting food cravings, the subjective power of food, dietary restraint, BMI, weight, somatic symptomology, anxiety, and depressive symptoms. Both treatments were also delivered over eight weeks.[9]

Our analyses revealed that over the eight weeks, both groups experienced significant reductions for food cravings, power of food, depression, anxiety, and weight, with these results remaining significant at the 6- and 12-month follow-ups. There were some differences observed in the post-intervention and/or six-month follow-up for dietary restraint and somatic symptoms.

The in-person format may have had a slightly stronger effect for dietary restraint than the online group, although the in-person group experienced a rise in somatic symptoms at the 6-month follow-up, increasing to preintervention levels before reducing once again at the 12-month follow-up to the post-intervention level. The online-group scores remained stable from post-intervention to 6 and 12 months for somatic symptoms.

Overall the majority of the aspects measured responded at a significant level for both versions of the program, and to date there is no other comparison of Clinical EFT in this way. It at least provides preliminary evidence that both styles of delivery are effective and valid.

SCHOOL STUDENT TRIALS

After our eight-week in-person and online trials, we featured in quite a few media stories. It turns out EFT is very interesting to journalists! A local school saw the story and asked if we could teach EFT to a group of students for healthy food choices.

We had 44 students aged 13 to 15 years who engaged in a six-week EFT program during school time.[10] This was with school, parental, and education-department approval. The students were randomly allocated to an EFT group or a wait-list group.

We taught the students how to use EFT for body-image concerns, resilience, and self-compassion. We also covered how to use EFT for drinking more water (and less soda), to increase their interest in exercise, and to help their sleep patterns. They did learn how to apply it to cravings, and also how to set goals.

After the wait-list demonstrated no changes occurred for them at all, they too received the six-week program. Then both groups were analyzed and followed up 11 weeks later (which was the end of the school year).

The EFT treatment resulted in a significant decrease in the consumption of *unhealthy drinks* (soda) after the six-week program, and this was still significantly low at 11 weeks follow-up. The group also reported a significant decrease in *unhealthy food choices*, and this too stayed changed at 11 weeks. We did have a mother e-mail the school to report that her 14-year-old son had requested cauliflower, and she could not quite believe it!

There were clinically valid decreases in the psychological distress scores (but not a statistical significance). One reason may have been that the EFT facilitators did not instruct the students to apply the tapping to various psychological symptoms specifically. Another is that it was a small sample size, and this would have affected the outcomes we saw.

In terms of self-esteem, results did indicate the students had significantly higher self-esteem and also self-compassion scores after the program.

This was a brief intervention and was limited by the end of the school year, meaning the follow-up period was short. However, it did highlight the utility of EFT to help with food and drink choices, and well as psychological concepts in teens.

THE BRAIN SCAN TRIAL

Since embarking on research in this field, I dreamt of conducting a brain scan trial involving tapping. Brain imaging is a powerful technique that is enhancing neuroscience research. Most conventional studies using fMRI (functional magnetic resonance imaging) are based on the BOLD effect, which is the term used to describe the increase in fMRI signal due to the change in blood oxygen and an increase in blood flow. BOLD fMRI has already been used to map how taste and odor occurs in humans and to study responses to pleasant and aversive stimuli.

Unfortunately fMRI studies are expensive, and the funding from traditional government sources was scarce. I didn't have access to a hospital that had the machine I needed. It seemed I had quite a few obstacles to overcome.

In late 2016 I became very clear about the set amount of money I needed to pay for the scans, and that I wanted the fMRI machine to be close to my university. I started to ask everyone I met if they had access to a machine; and while several people raised eyebrows, wondering what I was up to, I thought somehow it would get the word out.

I was right.

I received a telephone call on a Monday in late 2016 from a doctor at the local hospital. She was in a meeting with a range of health professionals, discussing the positive outcomes their chronic-pain patients were reporting with a technique called tapping. Ironically it was myself who had been teaching them. A nurse present mentioned I was looking for an fMRI machine to look at brain changes, and this doctor had access to one. She made the call. Did I want to use the machine?

Oh, and it was just a five-minute walk from my university to where the machine was located.

And that's how, in 2017, we conducted the world's first fMRI study of brain changes after EFT. For this first trial, we continued working with overweight and obese adults, but we'll have extended into chronic-pain patients by the time this book is published.

Previous neuroimaging studies have shown that in the brains of people who restrain themselves with food, emotional distress increases the reward value of food that is considered pleasant. This means when someone diets (using willpower or restraint) and becomes stressed or upset, then those foods they usually avoid appear *very* rewarding to them—and their brains reflect this effect.

We wanted to verify the brain activation (using fMRI) in overweight/obese adults as they looked at images of high-calorie food and also investigate the changes in the brain following EFT treatment to see how it matched their reported symptom improvements.

The Setup of the Program

The majority of participants who volunteered were female (86 percent), and chocolate was the most commonly chosen food craving to address for the group.

Fifteen overweight/obese adults were allocated to a four-week EFT treatment or control condition. They did not get a choice; and in the end, 10 received the EFT treatment and 5 did not. The university Human Research Ethics Committee gave ethical approval, and the trial was registered under the Australian New Zealand Clinical Trials Registry.

All of our participants needed to be at least 18 years of age; both genders were included. They needed to be at least overweight (i.e., BMI between 25 and 29) or obese (BMI greater than 30), and not currently receiving treatment (psychological or medical) for their food cravings.

Adults who were pregnant and known sufferers of diabetes (types I and II) and hypoglycemia were excluded due to possible impacts on food cravings. Because of the fMRI aspect of the study, participants could not have any metal implants (e.g., pacemaker); and everyone completed an MRI head-safety questionnaire prior to the first scan.

Everyone was scanned in the fMRI machine for the first time in the morning and while fasting. They were allowed to drink water and were asked to have a cup of coffee or caffeinated drink 30 minutes prior to attending, to stay stimulated.

While they were in the machine, they had to keep perfectly still. They wore a headset that allowed random repeating images of six high-calorie foods designed to engage parts of the brain to be projected onto the screen. This was a six-minute task, and they were asked to imagine eating or drinking the food and drink while they watched.

What Happened?

When we asked them to think about consuming the food and drinks on the images we presented on the screen, there was significant activation in the superior temporal gyrus (associated with cognition and thought) and the lateral orbito-frontal cortex, which is associated with reward.

After the first scans, the 10 adults allocated to the EFT group attended a four-week, eight-hour program identical to the original four-week program we ran. The control group did nothing and received no treatment at all.

At the end of the four weeks, everyone was scanned again in the same manner (first thing in morning, fasting, and with the same six food and drink images). There was a marked reduction in the BOLD response in the superior temporal gyrus and lateral orbitofrontal cortex for the EFT treatment group only. The control group showed continued activation in these areas.

You can see this in the sample scans included here. (For the images in high resolution and full color, please visit my website: www.petastapleton.com.) The highlighted areas are the areas that activated when the participants imagined eating or drinking the item in the pictures. The first scan has significant activity (before any EFT treatment) and is on the top in Figures 7A, 7B, and 7C. The post-treatment scan is on the bottom for each set, and they all have a remarkable absence of activity.

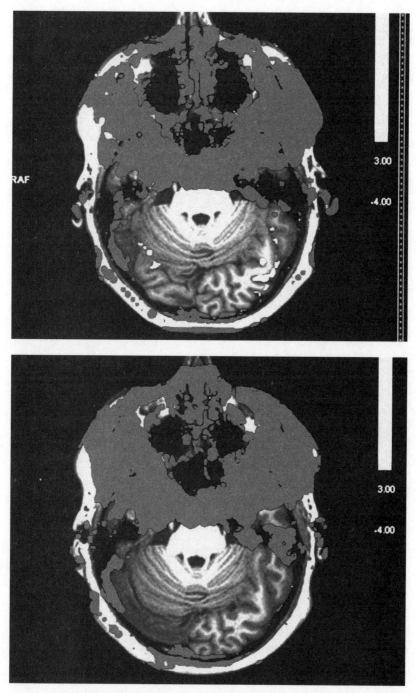

Figure 7A: Brain scan before and after EFT treatment

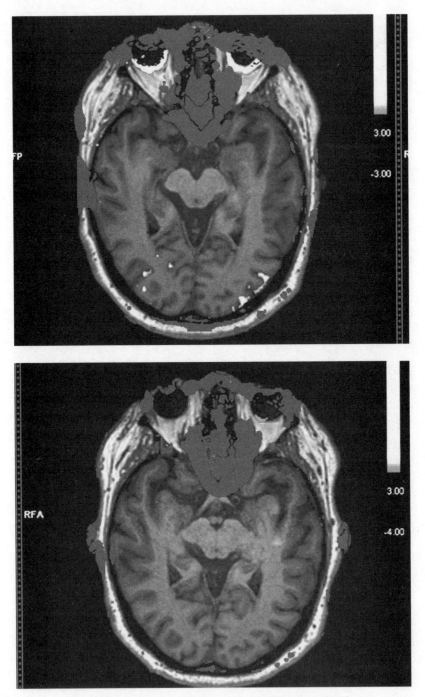

Figure 7B: Brain scan before and after EFT treatment

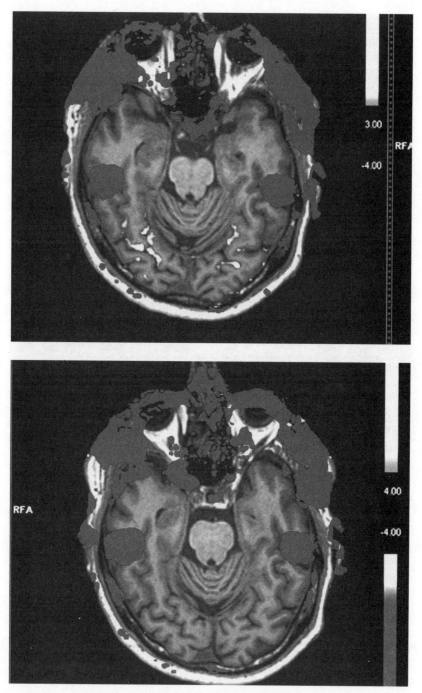

Figure 7C: Brain scan before and after EFT treatment

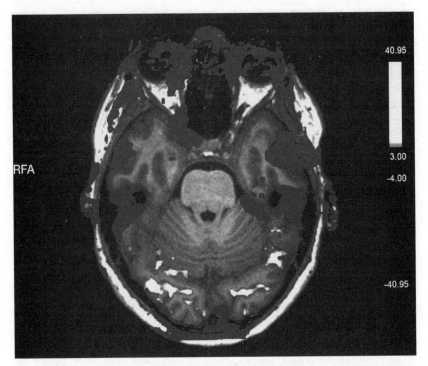

40.95

3.00

-4.00

RFA

-40.95

Figure 7D: Control-subject brain scan

I have included a scan of a control subject too, and you can see the level of activity is similar to the pre-treatment scans for the other participants. The difference was that they didn't receive any EFT intervention, and their scans looked the same at the post phase.

We also had participants complete our usual measures to examine food cravings and the like. The craving scores for carbohydrates over time reduced significantly between the EFT and control group (p=0.049), and the fast-food craving average difference over time also decreased significantly for the EFT group, in comparison with the control group (p=0.015).

In addition, the participants' power-over-food scores decreased significantly more for the EFT group, in comparison with the controls (p=0.019). It appeared the EFT treatment resulted in clinical symptom improvement that corresponded to a signal reduction in the two brain areas highlighted.

This was a pilot study and only included 15 adults; and in order to draw direct conclusions, future studies should be larger and longer in follow-up periods. It might also be preferable that individuals choose the most appropriate food images—ones that they would like to consume at the specific moment of the scan. We based the six images on our 10 years of trials, but individualizing them may be more powerful.

Nevertheless, this has been the first brain-scan study of EFT, and we would say it was a success. Future research will extend this study and also examine neural changes after EFT for chronic-pain patients.

After all, I owe that doctor who made the call.

FOUR-WEEK VERSUS EIGHT-WEEK TREATMENT

Because we have run two types of trials over the years (four-week and eight-week versions), we often wondered whether they were comparable or the longer one was more effective. Often patients vary in their response to treatment, including adherence, so it may be important to find out if shorter programs are as effective. This may then impact treatment adherence and completion.

So we have compared the two program lengths as they both measured the same variables.[11]

Outcomes indicated significant reductions in food cravings, subjective power of food, dietary restraint, body mass index, and weight for both interventions. There were no significant differences between the intervention groups in terms of the effect size of outcomes for the variables measured. Ultimately, the findings indicated that a briefer, four-week EFT intervention achieved *comparable results* to a longer, eight-week EFT program.

But for food cravings, the eight-week intervention produced effects that were maintained at the 6- and 12-month follow-up, while the four-week intervention did not maintain this effect at 6 months. The longer program may have resulted in improved cravings and is worthy of note for programs moving forward.

COMMON THEMES IN WEIGHT ISSUES

Because of all the research we have conducted in this area, we know there are certain things that absolutely need to be addressed if you are using EFT to target weight. This section will share the outcomes here as very practical steps if you are a practitioner working with patients, or ideas if you wish to apply them to yourself.

Common emotions individuals may have that trigger food cravings and food consumption include deprivation, abandonment, loss/grief/sadness, loneliness, emptiness, anxiety/stress, guilt, fear, anger, shame, wastage, and feeling inadequate/not good enough. We believe you need to address all of these with EFT.

Other examples participants offered included memories related to food (positive or negative) as a child; their first experience with using food to soothe a distressed feeling; and family patterns and beliefs around weight, food, and social acceptance.

These questions may assist in eliciting underlying emotional issues related to being overweight or obese, or having food cravings:

- How do you feel in your stomach when you eat a food that you crave?

- How do you feel in your stomach when you eat a food you don't crave?

- Seeing and smelling the food you crave, what do you feel?

- Imagine yourself throwing this food away. How do you feel?

- What's your first memory of eating the food you crave?

- As a child, were you given food to comfort you?

- What's your best memory that involves food?

- What's your worst memory that involves food?

The other significant issue that arose in our research was centered on wastage and disposing of craved foods. The most common emotional issues raised were *feelings of loss and guilt from food wastage.* Often participants highlighted messages from their childhood (e.g., "I feel guilty if I throw food away, because there are other people who are hungry"). Similarly, a feeling of guilt often resulted from an idea of being disloyal to a faithful friend (the food); and not seeking comfort in the food left participants with a sense of loss, emptiness, and unhappiness.

Feedback from the early food-craving trials highlighted many of the issues raised thus far. Interestingly, weight issues were often believed to be just that (devoid of any emotional content), as highlighted by a participant who chose not to engage in the food-craving trial:

> *Having perused your food-craving questionnaire, I have decided that my eating problems are not so much craving-related, but quantity-related! By that I mean both portion sizes and "doubling up" with either a second helping of the main course or following a main with dessert or fruit, etc. Added to that is the ever common "grazing" between meals! Compounding that is the fact that I have had Ross River virus for 15 years, meaning I experience pain and discomfort in my joints, particularly my feet, knees, and wrists (typical RRV symptoms). This limits the amount of exercise I do, even though I do physical work three days a week in my job. Thank you for the opportunity for me to give thought to my eating problems, and hopefully I can head in a different direction to achieve the results that I "crave"!*

The often-desperate pleas from would-be participants in the food-craving trials also flag a complex and deeply emotional weight journey:

> *My craving has been sugar for the past four years. I've put it down to hormones?? My GP said, "Just say no"!!! I'll be 53 in 11 days and weigh 95 kg at 168cm. Due to an accident, I have been unable to do a lot of exercise the last two years—yes, I'm using this and hormones as my excuse!! Wrong. I hope tapping*

those areas taught in the right way would help me shed the 20 kilos I have put on the past four years. Please can I be in your study???

. . . .

Finally I have read your article. I am not too overweight as I am about 170 cm and weigh about 69 kg, but I have constantly been up and down in my weight all my life. I diet and then go back eating. I absolutely love and live for food! I absolutely binge eat and love lollies, chocolate, etc. I cannot stop once I start. I get very depressed when I have to give them up. Could I please come to your trial as I would like to help you but also do something about this situation that I have battled all my life.

THE APPLICATION OF EFT FOR WEIGHT ISSUES: STAGE ONE AND TWO EFT

The remainder of this chapter is dedicated to practical setup statements and reminder phrases that may be used with clients with the basic technique, and that resulted from the clinical trials.

In stage one of our trials, we focused on food issues, underlying emotional issues, and related aspects. We then introduced choices and positive tapping in stage two, focusing on empowerment and installing positive reminder phrases. For example, if the problem is "fear of change," after tapping the SUD rating had decreased for the feeling and associated aspects, we followed with tapping on the same points with positive reminder phrases. These might include the following:

- I do want to change.

- They can handle it.

- I could be safe embracing this change.

- I love realizing my potential.

- I deserve [insert goal here].

- I appreciate all the abundance I have already.

- I appreciate who I am.

- I feel free to release this conflict once and for all.

In addition to positive phrases, participants included a choice or an "I choose" statement (described in Chapter 1), such as "Even though a part of me is afraid to change, I deeply and completely accept all of me, and I *choose* to succeed anyway." Some examples of positive or "I choose" setup statements can be reviewed in the examples of setup statements in this section.

Please note: While EFT has been reported to be of clinical use with other eating disorders (e.g., anorexia nervosa), the focus here is for its application for weight issues relating to being overweight and obese, although it could also be applied for eating disorders such as bulimia nervosa and binge eating disorder.

Situation: A food (usually junk) is regularly/frequently craved by the subject with a history of rarely or never resisting its consumption once the craving arises.

- **Examples of Setup Statements:**

- Even though I love sugary foods [or insert own food craving here], I completely accept myself.

- Even though I crave something sweet after meals [or whatever it is], I completely accept myself.

Reminder Phrases: This craving, my craving; love sugar; I crave this food; I love this food; desperate to eat this yummy . . .

Common Negative Belief or Thought: Afraid to let go of this problem; don't believe in myself

- **Examples of Setup Statements:**

- Even though I'm afraid to let go of this problem, I deeply and completely accept myself.

- Even though I don't believe I can reach my goal, I deeply and completely accept myself anyway.

- **Reminder Phrases:** Afraid to let go; afraid to change; don't believe in myself; can't reach my goal.

....

Feeling: Deprivation

- **Examples of Setup Statements:**

- Even though I feel deeply deprived, I deeply and completely accept myself anyway.

- Even though I can't eat like others, I deeply and completely accept this about myself.

- Even though when I restrict my intake, I feel deprived, I truly and sincerely accept myself.

Reminder Phrases: Feel deeply deprived; can't eat like others; feel deprived; feel restricted.

....

Feeling: Anxiety

- **Examples of Setup Statements:**

- Even though I can't stop feeling anxious/can't control my anxiety, I completely love and accept myself.

- Even though I am afraid that I won't know what to say and will make a fool of myself, I choose to accept myself anyway.

- Even though I'm afraid that I will lose control at [insert situation here], I completely love and accept myself anyway.

- Even though I know I tend to eat to relieve my feelings of anxiety or stress, I deeply and completely accept myself.

Reminder Phrases: Feeling anxious; can't stop being anxious; can't control my anxiety; I'm afraid I might make a fool of myself; I might lose control; I'm afraid; this fear; this anxiety; eat to relieve anxiety; eat to relieve stress; stressed.

. . . .

Feeling: Loneliness

- **Examples of Setup Statements:**

- Even though I feel this deep loneliness, I completely love and accept myself.

- Even though I feel lonely and completely empty inside, I love and accept myself.

- Even though I use food as my reliable friend because I feel so lonely, I completely love and accept myself anyway.

- Even though food keeps me company and stops me being aware that I am alone and afraid, I completely love and accept myself.

Reminder Phrases: I feel alone; lonely and empty; empty inside; completely alone; food has been my friend; food keeps me company; food stops my fear; I'm afraid to be alone; food stops me being lonely; food is reliable; this loneliness; loneliness.

. . . .

Situation: Exercise and motivation issues

- **Examples of Setup Statements:**

- Even though I loathe exercising, I deeply love and accept myself.

- Even though I feel fatigued and too tired to exercise, I choose to know that my energy levels will improve as I get fitter; I choose to be fit and healthy anyway.

- Even though exercise feels like punishment, I choose to know that it will help me, and I completely love and accept myself anyway.

- Even though I have no motivation to exercise, I completely love and accept myself.

- Even though I'd rather eat than jog, I completely love and accept myself.

- Even though exercise frightens me because I expect to get hurt or sore, I choose to know that it will help me, and I completely love and accept myself anyway.

- Even though I don't want to get too sweaty/hate getting sweaty, I completely love and accept myself.

- Even though I'm afraid I'll look too muscled and big, I choose to know that it's in my imagination, and I completely love and accept myself anyway.

- Even though I feel people think I look silly exercising, I choose to know that it's in my imagination, and I completely love and accept myself anyway.

Reminder Phrases: Loathe exercise; hate exercise; feel too tired; feel fatigued; choose to be fitter; choose to know I'll improve; it's too hard; feels like punishment; no motivation; no energy; I feel too tired; rather eat; hate jogging; don't want to; exercise frightens me; it's scary; it might hurt; hate getting sweaty; it feels yucky; too sweaty; exercise makes you big; too muscly; too big.

Situation: Given food as a comfort as a child; family issues

- **Examples of Setup Statements:**

- Even though my mother let me eat more biscuits/lollies/chocolate/junk food whenever I cried, I choose to love and accept myself.

- Even though my grandmother always overfed me to keep me quiet when I visited her, I choose to completely love and accept myself anyway.

- Even though my mother gave me ice cream to distract me from feeling sad and disappointed when my friends wouldn't let me play, I deeply and completely accept myself.

- Even though my dad started to buy me chips to make me feel better when I was disappointed about losing the football match, I deeply and completely accept myself.

- Even though I was fed [insert food here] to make me feel better when I was sick, I deeply and completely accept myself.

Reminder Phrases: [Insert food] when I cried; [insert food] made me feel better; Grandma and food; overfed to keep quiet; eat and be quiet; [insert food] to avoid disappointment; eat to avoid the feeling; [insert food] for comfort; [insert food] to handle disappointment; [insert food] and my dad; food to feel better; fed to combat sickness.

. . . .

Situation: Dislike of drinking water

- **Examples of Setup Statements:**

- Even though I dislike the taste of water, I deeply and completely accept myself.

- Even though I don't like drinks that have no smell, I deeply and completely accept myself.

- Even though I'd prefer to drink [insert beverage] than drink water, I deeply and completely accept myself.

- Even though I'm worried that drinking more water will mean going to the toilet too often, I deeply and completely accept myself.

- Even though drinking water is a nuisance to me, I deeply and completely accept myself.

- Even though drinking water doesn't excite me, I deeply and completely accept myself.

Reminder Phrases: Dislike the taste; smells horrible; hate the feeling in my stomach; I'd rather drink something else.

....

Situation: Using food to change mood

- **Examples of Setup Statements:** Even though I used food as entertainment and to stop myself feeling bored, I completely love and accept myself anyway.

- Even though I used food as security, I choose to accept myself anyway.

- Even though I overate to distract myself from [insert feeling or situation], I completely love and accept myself anyway.

- Even though I overate to avoid [insert feeling or situation], I completely love and accept myself anyway.

- **Reminder Phrases:** Food for entertainment; food to stop boredom; food for security; food makes me safe; food for distraction; didn't want to feel anything; food blocked the pain; overate to avoid; this avoidance.

....

Situation: Benefits or upside to staying overweight and not changing

- **Examples of Setup Statements:**

- Even though staying heavy/overweight/fat reduces the pressure on me so that people won't expect more, I deeply and completely accept myself.

- Even though staying overweight makes me feel invisible and safer, I choose to love and accept myself anyway.

- **Reminder Phrases:** Staying heavy; less pressure; it's easier; feels safer.

Situation: Negatives or costs to reaching a natural (ideal) body shape

- **Examples of Setup Statements:**

- Even though I need the distraction of overeating and hating myself, I choose to let this go and be slim anyway and completely love and accept myself.

- Even though I'm afraid of disappointing myself and others if I regain the fat, I choose to accept myself anyway.

- Even though I'll have no excuses anymore to not [insert activity here], I completely love and accept myself anyway.

Reminder Phrases: Need the distraction; need to hate myself; afraid I'll regain it; afraid I'll find it again; afraid I'll yo-yo; afraid I'll be back where I started; I'll be disappointed; [Insert name] will be disappointed in me; no more excuses; I can't hide behind excuses anymore.

Situation: Other negative consequences to reaching goal weight or body shape

- **Examples of Setup Statements:**

- Even though I can't afford new clothes, I choose to be slim anyway and completely love and accept myself.

- Even though I don't want to feel the pressure of keeping my new shape, I choose to be slim anyway and completely love and accept myself.

- Even though I won't be able to hide behind the extra fat anymore, I choose to completely love and accept myself anyway.

- Even though I resent having to maintain and be responsible for my control, I completely love and accept myself anyway.

Reminder Phrases: Can't afford new clothes; cost money; the pressure; it's too stressful; I'll feel trapped; can't hide away anymore; I'll be noticed; no excuses; scary; resentment; responsibility; no excuses.

TAKE-HOME POINTS

The application of EFT for weight issues is far-reaching and often complex. EFT can reduce immediate food cravings; EFT can target and eliminate negative or distorted body images; EFT can neutralize issues from the past that have led to overeating; and EFT can be used to target future situations that might trigger a relapse.

Everyday stress is often a factor in overeating. It is well known that EFT can help people manage this stress. EFT can confront and "loosen" the unconscious and conscious irrational beliefs individuals have about food, weight, and hereditary factors that may contribute to them being overweight. EFT can target and eliminate the negative or distorted body images that individuals hold about themselves, and can enhance a person's positive successful image of self.

EFT can be used to target future situations that might trigger a relapse, and can assist individuals in eliminating limiting beliefs about reaching their ideal weight and shape goals.

We have shown that the four-week, eight-hour program achieves almost identical outcomes to the eight-week program, and this may be important in situations where time is limited. And while an excellent advantage of using EFT is its precision in achieving change very quickly, the standout difference between the original four-week and eight-week food craving trials we conducted was the changes the more elderly participants received in the *later part* of the program.

It was often not until session seven or eight that "lightbulb" moments occurred or emotional release was achieved for those aged 65 and over. This may well be vital to remember when working with individuals who have had many years of ingrained behavior patterns and require more time to learn and accept the power of techniques such as EFT.

Our trials also showed a dramatic difference in brain activity after just four weeks of tapping for food cravings, and the online trial was able to achieve identical outcomes to those gained by attending in person. Ultimately the addition of EFT to any weight loss or maintenance program would not only be advisable—I would strongly suggest it is vital.

EFT FOR YOUNG PEOPLE AND STUDENTS

Children and teens do experience stress, but they may have a hard time expressing and articulating how they are feeling in a healthy way. How can we teach the children we love how to recognize, understand, and express their emotions in a self-empowering way? In addition, how can we help our children reduce stress, anxiety, and fear of failure?

Melinda, for example, was a bright and likeable 11-year-old, conscientious and careful in her schoolwork. However, while she liked school, and her teachers always loved her presence in their classes, she struggled with some aspects of learning. She was quite an experimental learner and liked to "feel" to learn.

This worked well for subjects where she could experiment (science) and even in the earlier years where mathematics may have been taught using physical counting blocks. But when it came time for spelling in the fifth grade, she couldn't find a way to learn the right spelling. Other students were able to visualize or memorize the words, but Melinda just couldn't.

She was very stressed by the end of the school year and miserably failed the final spelling test that was the benchmark for the next school year, receiving 45 out of 100. The teachers were concerned and raised the idea of her repeating the year with her parents.

This is not too uncommon a scenario for some students. Their learning style may not always match that of the teacher, and they appear not to be achieving. However, Melinda's mother was an EFT practitioner and knew she might be able to help. (We will come back to her in this chapter.)

FEAR AND FAILURE IN STUDENTS

Fear of failure and emotional difficulties are particularly common in high-achieving students. This often results in self-handicapping and defensive pessimism, which leads to failure or lowered academic achievement.[1] We know students who are engaged in the content they are learning have better retention and improved problem-solving skills.

But students often face barriers that prevent active-engagement learning, such as stress. Stress has the potential to affect memory, concentration, and problem-solving abilities, which can then lead to decreased student engagement and self-directed learning.

Fortunately we also know that higher levels of self-esteem and resilience are shown to protect against fear of failure and emotional difficulties, and predict improved academic outcomes in both high school and university students. However, few studies have investigated low-cost group-intervention methods aimed at improving self-esteem and resilience in students.

It turns out EFT is very effective for reducing anxiety, stress, and other emotional issues; and it works on both real and imagined stressors for children and teens. It can significantly increase positive emotions and self-esteem and resilience too, and decrease their negative emotional states. And interestingly, it is often easier to teach them, and they achieve faster results.

Let's start with the evidence for university student concerns.

THE RESEARCH FOR UNIVERSITY ACADEMIC ISSUES

A common area of focus in research examining university students has been that of test or exam anxiety. Have you ever felt nervous before a test or a performance? It turns out it is very common. This state of blanking out and freezing up, zoning out, or feeling so nervous that you can't get it together to respond to those questions you knew the answers to just last night severely affects 20 percent of students. Another 18 percent suffer these symptoms moderately.[2]

I have had a student standing in front of a tutorial class, ready to present on a topic as part of their assessment. And promptly faint. In front of everyone, just like that. Her brain was overwhelmed with the stress response and shut everything down. She did disclose an enormous fear of public speaking later that day, but she'd thought she could grit her teeth and get through it. Her brain thought otherwise.

The body's nervous system in overdrive like this doesn't do anything to help memory retrieval either! EFT has been studied for this type of thing in students and adults; and because the technique results in a calmer physical state, it usually helps with memory and better grades. It is also particularly quick—one study has shown public-speaking anxiety reduced significantly after just 15 minutes of EFT, with further significant reductions at 30 and 45 minutes.[3]

Test Anxiety

Psychiatrist Dr. Dan Benor and colleagues in 2009 conducted a pilot study of EFT and compared it to a Wholistic Hybrid derived from EMDR and EFT (called WHEE) and cognitive behavioral therapy (CBT). They were interested in how these three treatments would impact test anxiety in 15 university students (5 students in each condition). This was a pilot study, and while significant reductions in test anxiety were observed for all three treatments, more rapid benefits were observed in the experimental treatments (WHEE and EFT). Both WHEE and EFT achieved the same benefits as CBT did in five sessions, but they only took two sessions each to achieve it, potentially suggesting EFT and WHEE may have more rapid treatment effects. The students who received the experimental treatments were also observed to successfully utilize the skills learned and apply them to other stressful areas of their lives.[4]

EFT has also been compared to diaphragmatic breathing with solid outcomes. This type of breathing is often taught to people for anxiety and stress (it is breathing that is done by contracting the diaphragm). Researchers in the U.S. randomly assigned 168 university students to three groups: group 1 learned EFT for test anxiety, group 2 learned diaphragmatic breathing, and group 3 did not receive any treatment (control group).[5]

The researchers measured psychological symptoms, test-anxiety levels, and self-care behaviors before and after the two-hour lesson participants received. On a scale of 1 to 5, where 1 was "not at all," and 5 represented "extremely," students were asked how well they did in these areas:

- Eating a healthy, nutritionally balanced diet
- Getting adequate rest on a regular basis
- Getting a healthy amount of exercise each week
- Practicing healthy forms of relaxation on a regular basis

They were also asked to create a qualitative list of their particular issues that they believed contributed to their test anxiety, trouble studying, and less-than-optimal test performance. This list was used in the treatment they received.

Students also completed the Sarason Reactions to Tests (RTT) inventory, a 40-item questionnaire to assess self-reported levels of test anxiety. The higher the students' scores were, the greater their anxiety. The RTT measures four different components that typically interfere with test-taking success: test irrelevant thinking, bodily symptoms, tension, and worry.

The Symptom Assessment-45 Questionnaire assesses general psychiatric symptoms and was also used. Lastly, students completed the 10-item Westside Test Anxiety Scale. Six items of the scale assess impairment, and four items measure worry.

Groups 1 and 2 were asked to self-apply the technique they were taught for five minutes before any study session or exam, for a total of four weeks. They were followed up several weeks later at the end of the teaching semester.

The breathing group had a significantly higher increase in the self-care gain scores than did the tapping or control groups (there was no significant difference in the gain scores for these groups).

The breathing group also had a significantly higher decrease in the levels of test anxiety than the tapping or control groups. However, the tapping group did report a significant decrease in their levels of test anxiety, as compared with the control groups.

Overall, both the EFT and breathing groups had significant reductions in their symptoms, and the gains they made were still present at the end of the semester.

Anxiety actually increased in the participants in the control group.

Stress: A Comparison of EFT to Sham Tapping

Another study of 56 American university students wanted to examine EFT for stress and compare it to sham tapping.[6] The students were enrolled in a fourth-year thesis psychology program. They were randomly assigned to either the EFT (26 students) or sham group (30 students). For both groups, 69.6 percent were female, and 28.6 percent male, with ages ranging from 20 to 50 years old (average 23.4 years).

They were all assessed for nine common stress symptoms before and after a single 15-to-20-minute group session of 5 to 10 students.

They were asked to rate (within the past six months) if their sleeping or appetite had changed. On the day of the group, they were also asked to rate whether they were feeling physical tension, whether they were experiencing more emotional stress than normal, how worried or anxious they were about future events, whether they had difficulty taking deep breaths or concentrating on tasks, whether they were experiencing any physical pain, and whether today was a good day.

Participants in both groups then repeated statements from a script containing eight sets of stressful cognitions centered on feeling overwhelmed and hopeless, and ending with positive affirmations.

The EFT group tapped as per *The EFT Manual* points. The sham group used an identical procedure except that participants were taught to tap with their fingertips on sham points. These included the top of the hand, elbow, shoulder, forehead, stomach, knee, and thigh. Every effort was made to keep the two protocols identical with the exception of the body points.

Stress symptoms declined significantly more in the EFT group than they did in the sham tapping group. In the EFT group (26), symptoms declined 39.3 percent, whereas the sham tapping group had an 8.1 percent reduction. While Chapter 3 discussed the other comparison studies, this one showed that when all other components of treatment remain identical, *stimulation of actual points is superior to sham points.*

Public-Speaking Anxiety: Testing EFT and Generalization

Researchers in the UK have been interested to see if EFT as a skill would generalize to other areas taught.[7] In 2013 Dr. Elizabeth Boath and colleagues focused on comparing 47 male sports-science students aged 20 to 47 years with 43 females aged 26 to 59 years studying complementary alternative therapy (CAM). All were suffering from public-speaking anxiety.

Students were asked to rate their level of distress and to complete the Hospital Anxiety and Depression Scale (HADS). They were then given a brief 20-minute lecture that introduced them to EFT. Each group was guided through three rounds of EFT, focusing on their anxiety around their assessed presentation. Each round of EFT lasted approximately two minutes.

They were instructed that they could continue to use EFT anytime they wished to reduce their presentation anxiety. A reminder sheet summarizing the tapping points and giving example setup statements was made available to the students.

While this study was not focused on a clinically diagnosed population, interestingly their scores indicated a very anxious student body. Typically, a HADS score of 8 to 10 indicates a potential clinical issue that needs monitoring. Twenty-eight (60 percent) of the sports students scored 8 or above on the anxiety subscale before EFT compared with 23 (53 percent) of the CAM students.

In the sports students, the average anxiety subscale score reduced to below the clinical cutoff of eight after the EFT (average 7.24), whereas anxiety levels were still just within the clinical range for many of the CAM students (average 8.06).

Depression subscale scores were below the clinical cutoff point in both groups in the beginning; therefore there were no significant differences for either student group.

Overall, students experienced a significant reduction in self-reported anxiety, regardless of the group they were in, their age, or gender. EFT successfully reduced presentation anxiety in both groups. It did paint a picture that EFT may be generalizable.

The study openly acknowledged limitations. The HADS is not specifically designed to measure presentation anxiety, and the vast majority of students were white British in this trial. Whether the findings from this study of students in the Midlands of England can be generalized to other ethnic and cultural backgrounds still remains a question.

A Further Study on Public-Speaking Anxiety

These same researchers looked at 52 university students who were studying a research-methods subject and had to give a presentation.[8] It was known this always created anxiety among them. All the students attended a 15-minute EFT lesson where they applied tapping to their public-speaking fear.

They had their worry assessed using the HADS before and after the lesson (approximately 30 minutes), and were told they could use EFT anytime they wanted for their presentation, which was happening eight weeks later. Immediately after their presentation piece, 46 students were interviewed to find out who had used EFT beyond the 15-minute lecture.

Nineteen had used EFT for their presentation anxiety and 27 had not. Reasons for not using EFT included forgetting, feeling "silly" tapping in public, and uncertainty that they were doing it right.

Students who had used EFT actually received significantly higher grades than those who had not (p<0.01). There was also a significant reduction in their anxiety scores. The average anxiety scores before EFT (10.22) were well over the clinical cutoff point for anxiety; following the EFT intervention, however, they reduced to 7.83 (a nonclinical level). Depression was not affected at all as the baseline rates were normal.

The interviews indicated the students found EFT to be useful to enhance academic performance. Students found the skill calming and helped with focus:

> *Yes. I did it [EFT] in the car. It helped. I didn't sleep well last night—got a dry mouth and feel shaky, but not as bad as I usually am when doing a presentation. My legs are normally going, but they are alright today. It definitely took the edge off. I would definitely use it again. Used it for helping me to sleep and will use it again in future. — Kelly*

. . . .

> *Yes I usually go blank, I forget. And I used it to keep me focused today. I also used it when I first sat down and looked at the assignment. It did actually work. — Jacky*

. . . .

Yes, I did it before I came in and yesterday. It really helped me actually. It helped me to calm down. Helped my emotions—my anxiety, nervousness. Helped me to calm down really. It took the edge off the presentation. — Roberta

I have done it a few times for other things, for example when I am feeling a little bit worried . . . It was something to do while waiting outside. Tapped in the corridor! — Anne

Limitations did include that the lead researcher was not blind to treatment group, the students were aware that the authors were highly experienced, advanced EFT practitioners and that all had a strong allegiance to EFT. This may have influenced students' responses. However, the results do suggest a potential role for EFT as a brief group intervention to reduce presentation anxiety and potentially enhance academic performance.

THE RESEARCH ON HIGH SCHOOL STUDENTS

While much research is focused on students reducing negative feelings, EFT can also be taught for overcoming things like limiting beliefs that may act as a mental block for goals being achieved.

Goal Setting

We have taught this type of approach to 16-to-17-year-old high school students who were nearing the end of their schooling. Many of them had goals such as wanting to achieve a certain grade to gain entry into college or university or sporting goals.

One student we knew really wanted to be the school captain (leader) and represent the school the following year. But he needed to be voted in by his peers and teachers. He had a long list of reasons why this "couldn't possibly" come true—from not being popular enough among his peers to not being extroverted enough as a leader. We had him write down all the possible reasons that could be blocks to this goal coming true, he measured his SUD rating, and then we used EFT to systematically tap through them and reduce their intensity, one by one.

His list of why he might *not* become school captain included these reasons:

- No one really knows me, as I am quiet.

- I haven't been at the school for the whole time. (He'd come to the school the year before.)

- I don't know if I can give a good enough speech at the assembly where potential students vie for the position (for voting)

- I have never really won anything before, so why would I win now.

We used those exact statements and put them in the "Even though . . ." formula and tapped our way through them. We got to the end, and he felt fairly relaxed. I asked what his *belief* was now that he might become the school captain, and he said 10 out of 10! He didn't feel like there was any doubt left in him.

Obviously he still had to give the speech at the assembly later that year and then be voted in. I suggested he use tapping leading into that event, in case he was nervous or doubtful.

A year later I was talking to the school principal, having completely forgotten about the tapping with that student many months earlier. But I suddenly remembered and asked who was the school captain that year. The principal said, "You know, this unknown student just stood out, and he has been fantastic. It is _____." Of course I started laughing and told the principal he was one of the students we worked with on that very goal in the course we ran for the school a year prior.

Test Anxiety

In a large study, American researchers examined 312 high school students and identified 70 of them with high-level text anxiety using the Test Anxiety Inventory.[9] They randomly assigned these 70 students to a control group that received progressive muscle relaxation (PMR) techniques or to an experimental group that received EFT treatment. Every student engaged in a sample examination before receiving a single treatment session. The control group received instruction in PMR and the experimental group in EFT. At the end of the session, all students again completed a sample examination. They were then all asked to continue self-treatment at home.

After two months, all students were retested with the Test Anxiety Inventory, and 32 of the original 70 completed all requirements. Results showed a statistically significant decrease in the test anxiety scores of *both* the experimental and control groups. However, the EFT group had a significantly *greater decrease* than the PMR group ($p < .05$). The EFT group also scored lower on the Emotionality and Worry subscales of the Test Anxiety Inventory ($p < .05$). While the EFT group improved more on the sample examination after the intervention, both groups actually scored higher, and any differences were not statistically significant.

Ultimately while both groups reported a significant decrease in student anxiety, a greater decrease was observed for those who received EFT.

Mathematics Anxiety

A 2014 study investigated the effects of numerical cognition and EFT on mathematics anxiety among senior secondary students in three public secondary schools in Ibadan, Nigeria.[10] They had records of consistently low achievement in mathematics, and the researchers were able to obtain the academic records with school authority permission and cooperation.

There were 120 students included and a pseudo-dyscalculia scale was used to identify those with mathematics phobia. They also completed the Mathematics Anxiety Scale, the Mathematics Self-Efficacy Scale, and a mathematics achievement test.

Students were allocated to one of three groups: Numerical Cognition, EFT, or a control group. Numerical Cognition proposes students are more likely to find a solution to a problem when they concentrate on their successes rather than their failures. The trial occurred over 10 weeks during the school term.

The results showed the EFT intervention was more effective than the Numerical Cognition approach. It reduced students' mathematics anxiety more at post-test evaluation, especially among students with high mathematics efficacy.

Academic Stress in High-Achieving Students

My own research in high school students came about as a result of media attention we gained because of our food-craving trials. On the surface this doesn't seem related, but one of the main factors affected when you use EFT for food cravings is anxiety. We continually see a large reduction in anxiety when adults tap on wanting to eat a food they craved. So the media at the time was reporting this in stories.

A local school guidance officer made contact to enquire whether EFT would work just for anxiety in students. The answer was, of course, *yes*. And so we conducted the largest trial of 15-year-olds suffering academic stress to date.[11]

In total, 204 Year 10 (freshman) students from two Australian high schools participated: 80 were allocated to the EFT intervention group from one school, and 124 from the second school acted as a wait-list control (and they received the intervention at the end of the first group's course; both groups were demographically similar).

The average age of the students was 14.8 years, and more than 50 percent were female. All students were engaged in academically advanced programs, and all EFT treatment was delivered *in school time*, with parental and school permission (and ethical approval from the university and the government's Department of Education, Training, and Employment).

The students all received five weekly sessions of 75 minutes each during normal school hours and a booster session one year later. All students completed questionnaires about self-esteem, resilience, their perceived strengths and difficulties, and their fear of failure at the start of the program, at the end of the program, at six months, and at a year later.

The types of statements students used the EFT process on in the trial included common fears and beliefs raised by another Australian researcher who investigates these stressors in school students.[12] Examples included these statements:

- School is a waste of time.
- I can't do this.
- There's no point in trying.
- There's no way I can succeed.
- I might as well give up.

The students also learned to apply tapping for three barriers that are prominent for teens (this was important for the teens to want to use the technique beyond the trial and also at home in between sessions):

- Forgetting to tap.
- Doubting that EFT can or will work.
- Becoming confused or frustrated with EFT.

EFT was also used to target limiting beliefs and their application to areas such as academic and sporting performance (this appealed to them a great deal!):

- Success will make me stand out.
- Success will hurt my peer relationships.

- Success will put pressure on me to perform in future.

- I do not deserve success.

And finally, three other areas were addressed:

- Student's limiting expectations of themselves at school and in other areas of life

- Their perceptions of other people's expectations regarding their behavior and achievements (e.g., parents)

- Goal setting for the future, including doubts about achieving these goals

What was interesting was that the students' baseline resilience scores indicated the presence of anxiety levels commonly found in populations suffering from generalized anxiety disorder. The students' self-report measures indicated normal levels of self-esteem, however, so this was not impacted in the study. Overall what they did indicate as their main worries were self-perceived difficulties in life and a strong fear of failure.

The largest statistically significant change we saw was from the start of the program to a year later. *Fear of failure* was the most significantly affected variable, and students indicated in their survey 12 months later (compared with when they started the trial) that this was the most impacted area in their lives. *This meant they did not feel anywhere near the same fear of failure as before they started the tapping.*

We noted that most students did not continue tapping beyond the end of the trial. However, the results achieved indicated a five-week EFT program had the potential to assist students' perceived difficulties and impact their fear of failure and remain stable a year later (the memory reconsolidation theory may be the answer here). The potential improvements in student functioning, the ease of teaching EFT in a group, and the cost-effectiveness suggest that further research is warranted; but EFT may offer students significant benefits with low risks and time demands, at relatively low financial cost to schools.

EFT FOR GIFTED CHILDREN

Tapping with children can be a fairly straightforward process, as they tend to be less complicated than adults in their concerns, and are often open to the process. It is suggested that gifted children may experience additional stressors due to their unique characteristics, and they may suffer from higher levels of stress due to perfectionistic tendencies, heightened sensitivity, social challenges, and additional external pressures.

This is an area that is largely under-researched, however, as it requires parental or guardian consent and needs to be guided by stricter ethical standards. There are few published trials on EFT specifically for children to date, but one study by Dr. Amy Gaesser and colleagues stands out by focusing on gifted children and teens.[13]

This study took place in 10 schools (8 public and 2 private; 4 high schools and 6 middle schools) in two northeastern states in America. There were 63 high-ability students (aged 10 to 18 years) who were identified as anxious. There were 18 males and 45 females, and all were within the top 15 to 20 percent of their peer groups academically. Everyone completed the Revised Children's Manifest Anxiety Scale-2, and all scored at moderate-to-high anxiety levels.

Students were randomly allocated to an EFT group, a CBT group, or a wait-list control group (all groups had 21 students). Those students in the CBT or EFT treatment groups received three individual sessions of treatment. Sessions occurred over a five-month period, with most occurring not less than one week or more than two weeks apart.

The EFT group showed significant reductions in their anxiety levels compared with the wait-list control group; and while the CBT students showed a reduction in anxiety too, they did not differ significantly from the EFT students. What this meant was the EFT was comparable to a gold standard treatment like CBT and could achieve the same outcomes. Larger trials are necessary, but at least the evidence is promising.

I hope we continue to see published trials in younger children, and we have begun several of these in Australia. Encouraging a skill such as tapping to be a normal part of dealing with stress when a child is young may result in differences in diagnoses later in life.

NOTES FROM A PRACTITIONER: ANXIETY IN HIGH-PERFORMING STUDENTS

EFT practitioner Julie Vandermaat shared with me how the application of tapping to a teenage student trying to achieve perfection can have a real impact.

"Alex" was 15 years old. He was referred by his mother, as she was concerned about how unhappy and negative he was feeling. Alex was academically bright and good at sports, but socially he had had difficulties for years.

In the first session, Alex immediately said what was wrong with him, and why he was feeling unhappy and negative. He said "I am not attractive, I know that much. I am undervalued at school. I am insecure, as I don't have a good friendship group. I am unwanted. I have a few friends, but I don't socialize well with other people. I never make the right choice."

He stated he was not perfect, not even close. When asked what percentage of perfect he thought he was, he said, "About 2 percent." He felt he was never going to reach his goal of being 100 percent perfect, and he estimated that he felt self-conscious about 85 percent of the time. His lack of confidence, combined with these associated issues, bothered him 10 out of 10.

Alex said what he wanted was to be happy, to feel accepted, and to feel okay about being himself around others. He thought his problems started at the end of the sixth grade, when most of his childhood friends went to a different high school. He reported that he had been feeling negatively about himself for three years. He had tried changing schools, but this made the problem worse.

After numerous rounds of EFT, Alex became aware that he had a lot of unexpressed grief and sadness over the loss of those good friendships in the sixth grade. He reflected that this was the last time he felt like he could really be himself and that people accepted him as he was. He shed a few tears as he talked about missing those friends, and about how painful it was to feel like he was never going to feel that level of acceptance again.

They finished the session with Alex feeling 6 out of 10 on the SUD rating scale.

....

At the next session a week later, Alex had only positive changes to report. His self-consciousness had reduced to 70 percent, then 50 percent by the end of that session. He rated his lack of confidence as 5 out of 10, and it came down further to 3.5 out of 10. He felt about 30 percent perfect, and said he had made some great new friends.

He was happy to do some more EFT, and he knew it worked now.

After session one, Alex's mother said she felt like she had a "new boy" in the house. She was astounded at how quickly EFT had helped him become so happy and relaxed. Alex rated himself to be self-conscious less than 10 percent of the time.

After completing several sessions of EFT, Alex continued to improve. His lack of confidence only bothered him 0.5 out of 10 now. His mood was 9 out of 10, and he said he now had better thoughts, like "I am good, I am accepted and likeable." He stated he was no longer so harsh on himself and was learning to accept himself and his appearance more.

Alex said he hated school before EFT, but was now enjoying learning more.

He happily reported he had created a new basketball team with all his new friends in the year above him. When asked if there was anything left to tap on he replied, "No, I've fixed all my problems now."

Weeks later, Alex's mother reported he was still feeling really happy with himself and still had the new group of friends.

THE EMOTIONAL DISTRESS OF LEARNING DISABILITIES

There has been a case study completed on how EFT can be used for dyslexia (a learning condition which is evident in reading comprehension, spelling, and writing). Often the condition causes a child emotional distress as well. While this study is a single case study (often useful as the basis for larger trials), it is a starting point to learn what works and what doesn't and is worthy of note.

Fiona McCallion, a London therapist, worked with a woman in her 20s who suffered dyslexia and had sequencing, disorientation, and emotional feelings attached to it. They had three sessions and addressed all of these areas with EFT. They started with past memories of teachers who had ridiculed her in class when she was younger.[14]

The second session focused on two specific incidents involving two teachers at school. One was a math class where she was not given the marks for correct answers because she couldn't explain the method she used to arrive at them. While she received marks for an incorrect answer (based on the method used), when she got the answer right, she got zero points because she couldn't explain the method. You can imagine how confusing this might be for a child.

By the end of the three EFT sessions, the client was able to read easily and fluently and understand sentences. The disorientation associated with the client's dyslexia had also reduced significantly to a point where it was no longer an issue. Using tapping to explore and assist with emotional distress attached to learning concerns is therefore highly recommended, and the applications in these settings may be boundless.

TRAINING TEACHERS IN BEST PRACTICES FOR EFT WITH THEIR STUDENTS

There has started to be interest in the school systems for teachers to be trained in delivering EFT as a daily stress-regulation skill. One-off trials may not be the most effective dissemination of the technique; and given teachers do not typically deal with trauma-related issues in a classroom, using tapping as a daily tool for stress and worry may be very useful.

Some programs are emerging designed to give teachers, school guidance counselors, psychologists, and parents an effective tool to help students overcome stress, anxiety, and behavioral challenges in the classroom on a daily basis. The idea of using tapping in classrooms for everyday anxieties (e.g., nerves before an exam, excess tiredness after lunch) is proving to be a better option.

The following are the types of things teachers are using EFT for in the classroom:

- To reduce stress, anxiety, fear of failure, and procrastination
- To help students improve academic performance for national exams and assignments
- To help students recognize, understand, and express their emotions
- For friend issues, anger, bullying, and self-harm (although school counselors may do more of this)
- To help students set and achieve goals
- To help reduce their own levels of stress and overwhelm as teachers
- To increase their own and students' happiness, energy, and sense of well-being

Tapping in the Classroom® as a training for teachers was developed out of our own school trials. The level of interest we were receiving worldwide indicated teachers wanted to learn this skill, but Australia was a bit far to travel!

The development of our online teacher training took some time, but it is now 100 percent online and self-paced. It is an eight-module training designed to give teachers the skills to help students do the following:

- Recognize and understand their emotions

- Discover how to become confident, resilient, and adaptable

- Improve well-being, self-esteem, and academic success

It is based on our clinical-trial research and designed to be understood and applied by anyone new to EFT or tapping. Online support continues after the training, in a dedicated forum space.

The training is a combination of movie files with instruction and application of EFT; videos of students tapping to watch and learn of their experience; practical exercises to do during the training and in between modules; and example tapping scripts, worksheets, handouts, and sample letters for parents and school staff.

To learn more, please visit: https://evidencebasedeft.com/tapping-in-the-classroom.

EFT AND ATHLETIC IMPROVEMENT

Comparing EFT with Standard Coaching in College Basketball

Dr. Dawson Church has completed research with 26 athletes using EFT.[15] The first was a randomized study with high-performance men's and women's Pac-10 college basketball team members. A total of 14 males and 12 females participated.

Everyone engaged in a warm-up standard to the teams' processes lasting 10 minutes and consisting of stretches and running.

They then performed 10 free throws, and two groups of three jumps (six jumps in total). The vertical height of the jumps was measured using a Probotics jump pad, which electronically records and displays jump height in tenths of an inch.

The athletes were then randomized by an independent research assistant into two matched groups, based on the average height of the second group of three jumps. During the study they were instructed to practice free throws, run, dribble, do vertical jumps, and generally stay warmed up.

One group then received 15 minutes of EFT. A participant was taken into a private office and taught EFT for 10 minutes on their own. They then went back to the court, performed three vertical jumps, and returned to the treatment room for an additional session lasting 5 minutes (in total receiving 15 minutes of EFT instruction). After this, they returned to the court to perform three final jumps and a posttreatment set of 10 free throws. Every athlete did this individually until the whole group was finished.

The control group received 15 minutes of inspirational basketball tips and techniques but no EFT.

The EFT team members improved on average 20.8 percent in free throws, compared with the control group who *decreased* on average 16.6 percent in free-throw ability. Interestingly, free throws increased an average of 2.6 percent for females in the EFT treatment group, while the control group *decreased* an average of 22.2 percent. There was no treatment group difference for males.

Vertical jump height wasn't affected at all, but given it was only a 15-minute EFT session, which still achieved significant results, it would be worth replicating this with a longer time frame to see what could be achieved!

Comparing EFT with Standard Coaching in Soccer

In soccer, two female English soccer teams (26 players in total, aged 15 to 30 years) engaged in an EFT session to improve goal-kicking ability or normal soccer coaching.[16] They all participated in warm-up exercises and completed a series of penalty goal attempts. The EFT group received a 10-minute session designed to match the basketball study outlined above to try to verify the results of brief EFT, and then attempted an unchallenged soccer goal from 50 feet away (as if for a "dead ball").

The results revealed a significant improvement in goal-scoring ability from the dead-ball situation following the brief EFT session. The study also showed a statistically significant difference between the two groups that the authors hypothesized might have related to a decrease in associated anxiety levels for the EFT group.

Traumatic Memory in Young Women's Volleyball

Church and Darlene Downs, D.D., have also looked at sports confidence in athletes who had a traumatic memory related to their sports performance.[17] Athletes were assessed on their level of distress when asked to recall either an emotionally troubling memory in which their "team did not win" or their "worst experience with a coach." They were excluded if their score was less than 3 on a Likert scale (ranging from 0: *minimal distress* to 10: *maximum distress*).

Participants were 10 female volleyball athletes (aged 19 years on average) who had academic scholarships based on their sports abilities. They had played volleyball for nine years on average. All women completed the State Sport Confidence Inventory and the Critical Sport Incident Recall Survey, and rated their distress on a SUD scale. They were measured at 30 days before the intervention, 15 days before, and just prior to the EFT session.

Athletes' pulse rates were measured at every time point as well with the Insta-Pulse 107, a portable handheld device that measures electrocardiogram rhythm and displays a four-heartbeat average. They also completed all assessments immediately after the EFT intervention and 60 days later.

Participants received an individual 20-minute EFT session where each athlete focused on her description of the traumatic memory (i.e., of her team not winning or of her worst experience with a coach).

Significant improvements in both the emotional and physical components of sports performance were seen after the session, and all improvements were maintained 60 days later. The pulse rate did not show significant reductions immediately after EFT but did show a significant reduction at follow-up.

While the sample size was small and all female, and there was no control group, the study still highlighted the possibility of EFT's ability to impact athletes' levels of confidence and distress, and possible future performance outcomes. Let's turn to another sporting area.

NOTES FROM A PRACTITIONER: OTHER CHILDHOOD CONCERNS

Most of the research discussed here focused on children and teens at school; however, EFT is used for many issues outside of academic ones. This account shared with me by Magda Mesquita in Portugal highlights how effective tapping can be for other childhood concerns. The second study, by Australia practitioner Desley Murphy, indicates that sometimes children need to tap on dealing with adults in their life.

Case Study: 10-Year-Old Sam

The client's mother came to the first session with Sam, her 10-year-old son, and she said he suffered from fecal incontinence. This had been a huge problem for a few years, ever since kindergarten. She reported that she had taken her son to psychologists, and he had taken medication prescribed by a doctor, but never got any results.

The mother reported she made Sam spend 10 minutes in the toilet every day, to see if it changed his bowel-movements habits, because sometimes he couldn't control himself at school.

As a result, his schoolmates made fun of him. She described Sam as introverted, which made it difficult for him to make friends with anyone.

As his mother talked about this issue and about him, Sam sat quietly and looked embarrassed by the conversation, refusing to comment or add any information.

Magda explained the nature of EFT and asked Sam if he was willing to try those "magic fingertip touches" on himself, and he agreed. Magda asked the mother to leave before beginning to teach tapping to Sam.

Magda told Sam there was even a way of addressing the issue without him having to talk about it. He listened very attentively. She asked him to describe this situation with just one or two words, and he said in a low voice, "This problem." Magda asked him to tell her how he felt about "this problem," and he said, "I feel bad," and then "I feel shame." She asked for the SUD level, and he answered 10 out of 10. She asked him if he could locate those emotions in his body, and he said face and head.

They tapped for a few rounds on "this problem" with the words "Even though I have this problem that makes me feel so bad and ashamed, I'm a really good boy." As the intensity of the shame came down to a 6, Magda asked Sam if there could have been anything that had happened in his childhood that might have contributed to this problem. He said, "Something happened in kindergarten when I was four years old. I felt very ashamed, and they made fun of me; I felt so sad." As he said this, he started crying. So they tapped on "Even though they made fun of me because of what happened, I am still a great kid." He refused to give out any details, so they just kept on tapping on the sadness and shame that the event brought up for him.

At the end of the session, Magda tested for the intensity of "this problem," and he said it was a 2. He looked relieved and more relaxed.

At his second session, Magda asked Sam how he had felt after the first session, how things were regarding "that problem." He said he had felt better. He was still shy, and he shrank his body as he talked. He said it was difficult to talk about it; he felt embarrassed.

She asked him how embarrassed he was on a scale from 0 to 10, and he said, "Ten." They started tapping right away: "Even though I'm too embarrassed to talk about it, I'm a really good kid." After the intensity came down to a more bearable 5, Magda asked him if he could remember any incident in which he might have felt that much embarrassed.

He gave it a title: "A bad day," and he rated the intensity at 7 out of 10. When asked to say how he felt about it, he said, "Ashamed" (SUD level 10). They tapped on the title of the story for a couple of rounds, and the 10 came down to a 5. He then felt comfortable enough to talk about it. He said it was in the fourth grade. It was the end of the school day, and they were packing their things in the classroom to go home, "and then it happened, and my classmates told the teacher—I just wanted to kill them!"

They tapped on the anger he felt in his head, as well on the aspects that came up:

"Everybody heard."

"They were whining about me."

"A girl whined about me to the teacher (girls are always whining)."

"She said I smelled bad."

"I couldn't do anything about it."

The initial intensity of 10 came down to a 0. Sam said, "I don't feel ashamed about this anymore, it doesn't bother me anymore."

. . . .

At the next visit, Sam walked into the office smiling and showing a much more confident body posture. Magda asked him how he felt, and he said with a big smile, "It's working! I feel much better! I've stopped doing it in my pants at school."

Sam retold the whole sequence of events from the sessions, without hesitating or showing embarrassment. He even mentioned things he had not talked about before. After what had happened in the classroom, Sam left to go and change his pants; and when he came back, his classmates made fun of him. He said, "They shouldn't have done that. It could have happened to anyone," and he was quite calm talking about it. He finished by saying, "When I am well, one day, I imagine I will feel like a normal person, and everything is going to change. My classmates will forget about all of this; I will forget about this; this will no longer be a problem."

This was quite remarkable to see.

This was the last session Magda had with Sam. He never had any incidents at school after three sessions; and after a six-month follow-up, his mother reported that he was a completely different boy, and the issue was no longer an issue. It had "completely gone."

Case Study: Five-Year-Old Thomas

Madonna bought her five-year-old son, Thomas, for an EFT session with Desley because he did not like school. After playing with some LEGO bricks on the floor with Thomas, Desley asked him to tell her his favorite thing about school. He said, "Reading, but we read the same boring words." According to his mother, he was a bright child who had a love of learning and was squashed by his teacher, who saw him as disruptive and rude for saying he was bored.

Desley said, "So you want to read different things."

Thomas said, "Yes, but Mrs. Stone said I have to read the same words as everyone else." He then said, "Mrs. Stone was very mean." His cheeks were red, and his brow furrowed, so Desley took those nonverbals as a 9 or 10 in intensity.

Desley said, "It sounds to me like you are pretty angry with Mrs. Stone, am I right?" The boy nodded. He seemed overwhelmed, so Desley did not ask him to measure his anger.

She asked him if he wanted to do some tapping to see if they could help him feel happier about learning new words. He agreed.

They tapped "Even though I am angry at Mrs. Stone for not letting me read new words, I am a good kid." They tapped through the points using the phrase "angry at Mrs. Stone."

Thomas's cheeks became very flushed as they tapped. At the conclusion of the session, he said, "Mummy, I felt a hot wind go up my cheeks, and all my anger at Mrs. Stone flew away." He was visibly happy and relaxed—actually excited.

Two weeks later his teacher called his mother aside and said that she was happy to report that Thomas had really settled into school. She said she couldn't explain it, but he seemed happier and more cooperative. She said even his handwriting had changed. She produced two samples of his writing: one from two weeks prior, scrawling and messy, and his work that day, neater and more legible. She was amazed at the visible difference.

This case was actually many years ago. Ironically, Thomas went on to be the dux (the highest-ranking student) of the school; and at the awards ceremony, he made a speech in which he thanked his teachers and said, "Even though Mrs. Stone and I locked horns in the first grade, we became friends."

Mrs. Stone was sitting in front of the mother and turned to her and said, "You should be very proud of your son." She was!

TAKE-HOME POINTS

As you can see from the case studies, there are so many applications of EFT for children and youth. While I have always worked clinically in the weight space, and my EFT research has been the same, the ability to work with this next generation has been a blessing. Teaching them a way of being able to calm themselves, achieve their goals, and handle stress may result in a very different world in decades to come. They also have a tool to release distress they may be carrying from years gone by.

We have now embarked on several whole school projects in Australia, and every teacher in every classroom has learned EFT and is using it daily. The students range from 5 to 13 years old.

We are tracking them for the next seven years to document the outcomes. Our aim is to make tapping a normal activity to do when you feel overwhelmed or stressed as a student. Teachers are benefitting as well!

The opportunity to write *EFT for Teens*, a book especially for teenagers to read and learn tapping in the privacy of their own bedrooms, has also been a journey down memory lane.[18] I can only imagine what life would have been like as a teen if I had known tapping. Now it is a joy to see my own daughters teach their friends and take it for granted as a stress-reduction tool!

Remember Melinda from the opening of this chapter? You may recall that she was failing her spelling. Her mother was an EFT practitioner and offered to help with her daughter's rising stress and worry. They did not focus so much on the actual spelling of the words on the master list, but instead tapped with statements related to letting the teacher down, feeling stupid, and not wanting to repeat the class another year.

After an hour of tapping, Melinda said she felt much calmer, and they stopped. Over the next week, her mother helped her review the spelling words and practice them (e.g,. with her eyes closed and spelling out loud). This strategy had never occurred to Melinda, but she found it helped her focus.

Ten days after the failed test, Melinda again took the spelling exam. She achieved 65 out of 100 and was on her way to the sixth grade! She has continued to tap for her worries.

THE IMPACT OF EFT ON FURTHER CONDITIONS

Tapping has been researched across many other conditions besides those already highlighted. However, often they are single studies, which are yet to be extended or replicated. Nevertheless, they do showcase the other areas starting to emerge.

A recent systematic review by one of my doctor of philosophy graduates, Dr. Mahima Kalla, examined EFT for enhancing physical, mental, and emotional health of people with chronic diseases and/or mental-health conditions.[1] She examined specific changes occurring in the physical body as a result of administering EFT (e.g., changes in cortisol levels, reduced clumping in blood cells, or a reduction in somatization) or when people reported emotional and mental-health benefits immediately and at a later follow-up time.

The review suggested that EFT can potentially be an effective supportive-care method for patients who need to manage psychological stress and stress symptoms on an ongoing basis because of a health condition.

Dr. Kalla also interviewed eight EFT practitioners to explore their use of EFT to support chronic-disease patients.[2] All interviews were transcribed verbatim, and data was analyzed using interpretative phenomenological analysis methodology (this is a way of seeing how a given person, in a given context, makes sense of a phenomenon such as a major life event).

She proposed that chronic-disease patients may benefit from holistic biopsychosocial, patient-centered health-care approaches, and that EFT offers this potential.

With this in mind, this chapter highlights the EFT studies that have focused on mental and emotional concerns as well as physical and physiological conditions.

PHOBIAS

Phobias are an unreasonable and often irrational fear that can cause avoidance (of the feared object/situation) and even panic. They are classified as an anxiety disorder. Anyone who has ever experienced the depth of fear that is associated with a phobia will know how difficult they are to overcome.

Phobia of Small Animals

The first research into phobias using tapping was by Australian practitioner Steve Wells in 2003.[3] He and his team evaluated EFT for reducing specific phobias of small animals. There were 35 individuals with a fear of small animals randomly allocated to an EFT intervention or a diaphragmatic breathing (DB) intervention. They all met the diagnostic criteria for a specific animal phobia.

The average age of the participants was 39.6 years (range was 19 to 72 years), and the average number of years suffering the phobia was 20. All adults completed the following measures prior to beginning their treatment:

- *A behavioral approach task (BAT):* This was designed to measure the participants' level of avoidance, seeing how close they would allow themselves to get to the feared animal. There were eight measurement points scored from 1 to 8 according to the point reached by the participant: (1) outside the room, door closed, and (2) outside the room with door open (six meters from stimulus animal). The next six points were inside the room, at the following distances away from the feared animal: (3) five meters; (4) four meters; (5) three meters; (6) two meters; (7) one meter; (8) directly in front. Participants were not encouraged to move closer to the animal at any time.

- *A fear questionnaire:* A modified form of the "brief standard self-rating for phobic patients" was used to measure phobic symptoms and change.

- *A subjective units of distress (SUD) rating when imaging the animal (SUD Imagined).* This consisted of a 10-point scale ranging from 0: no fear/distress to 10: intense/unbearable fear/distress. Participants were asked to give a SUD rating indicating how they felt when they imagined their phobic animal "here, right now." They were asked to rate how they felt at this moment, not how they imagined they would feel. SUD ratings were also recorded at each step taken on the behavioral approach task.

- *Pulse rate:* A research assistant took pulse rate manually following completion of demographic data, and once again at the point at which the client voluntarily stopped on the behavioral approach task.

- *Confidence rating:* Participants indicated during the pretreatment assessments how confident they were that their as-yet-unidentified treatment would work on an 10-point scale, from 0: not at all confident to 10: absolutely confident.

Both groups then received 30 minutes each of their respective treatment (they were all individual sessions). Twenty-one participants (12 in the EFT condition and 9 in the DB condition) took part in a six-month follow-up. The remaining could not be contacted.

For the EFT sessions, the full version of EFT (covering 12 acupoints) was used for the first three rounds of treatment, and a shortcut version (7 points) was used for the remainder. The deep breathing condition was designed to parallel the EFT condition, and the main difference was the fact that EFT participants tapped on acupoints, and DB participants used controlled breathing as their intervention (without a self-acceptance statement).

The EFT participants improved significantly more than the DB subjects in behavioral and subjective distress measures pre- to post-treatment; and while both conditions showed a significant decrease in pulse rate, there was no difference between them.

Improvements in the behavioral measure were also enhanced at the six-month follow-up for the EFT participants. There was also evidence that the improvements in the subjective distress measures were maintained in that they did not return to baseline levels. However, the superiority of EFT over diaphragmatic breathing dissipated somewhat at the follow-up point. The authors attribute this in part to the small sample size.

A. Harvey Baker and Linda S. Siegel did a partial replication and extension with the Wells phobia study in 2010.[4] They followed a similar protocol but added in a control group that was missing from the original trial. Individuals with an intense fear of small animals were assigned to a single 45-minute EFT intervention, supportive interview, or no-treatment control group.

Overall, significant decreases in fear of small animals were observed for those who received the EFT intervention only, with no change observed for the individuals who received no treatment or the supportive interview.

One year and four months later, the significant effects observed in the EFT group were maintained and continued to be superior to the other two conditions.

Both sets of findings from these phobia studies lend support for the effectiveness of tapping in the treatment of intense fear, and it appears to last over time. Both studies also indicated that the outcomes were achieved in *less than an hour* of EFT treatment.

Claustrophobia

Researchers wanted to investigate the effects of tapping for claustrophobia sufferers, in particular on its physiological effects.[5] Claustrophobia is the intense fear of being enclosed in a small space or room and unable to escape, and it causes severe distress for sufferers. For this study four claustrophobic and four normal individuals were recruited. This was a small study, but often these are better to conduct as pilot studies when the nature of the condition is complex.

The claustrophobic sufferers were measured with the State-Trait Anxiety Inventory; physiological measures of EEG, EMG, heart rate, respiration rate; and measures of the electro-conductance within the acupuncture meridians.

The results when compared with normal individuals showed that a 30-minute tapping treatment appeared to create reduction in EMG for the trapezius muscle (one of the major muscles of the back, it is responsible for moving, rotating, and stabilizing the shoulder blade and extending the head at the neck), changes of EEG theta wave activity, and changes in the electrical conductance between acupoints along a meridian pathway. The measures pre- and posttreatment on the anxiety inventory for the tapping group were significantly lower even two weeks later.

Specific Phobias

Finally, another pilot of 22 students with significant phobias of specific feared situations or objects has been conducted.[6] More than half of the sample was female (15 people, 68 percent)

with an average age of 20.8 years. They were predominantly His-
panic (16 people, 73 percent), in addition to Caucasian (5 people,
23 percent).

They all scored at least 8 out of 11 on an intensity scale for
their phobia, and these included fear of heights, snakes, darkness,
needles, and cockroaches.

Everyone was randomly allocated to either EFT or a deep-
breathing group; however, it had a crossover design so that the
deep-breathing students also received the EFT treatment afterward. All students were measured with a behavioral approach test
(BAT), SUD, and the Beck Anxiety Inventory (BAI).

The BAT varied for each phobia:

- *Fear of heights*: Participants were taken to the university stadium, which contained 38 bleachers, and asked
  to go up next to the outside guardrail, where they
  could clearly notice the height. It was measured as one
  bleacher (3 percent) to 38 bleachers (100 percent).

- *Snake phobia*: This was conducted in the university ser-
  pentarium with an observation room containing over
  20 terrariums with live rattlesnakes. This was scored
  from being no less than seven feet from the observation room (14 percent) to being inside the observation
  room, two feet away from the snakes (100 percent).

- *Darkness*: This was done in an office with no light and
  involved walking toward the dark room but stopping
  before standing in front of the closed door (14 percent)
  to being inside the dark room, with the door completely closed for at least five seconds (100 percent).

- *Needles*: This ranged from seeing the researcher (sitting
  approximately five feet away) hold a syringe inside a
  plastic package (14 percent) to seeing the researcher
  simulate an injection (rubbing alcohol on arm and
  placing the needle right next to the arm; 100 percent).

- *Cockroaches*: A live cockroach was in a jar, and the test ranged from standing three feet from the jar (20 percent) to holding the jar and opening the lid (100 percent).

Tapping significantly reduced the students' phobia-related anxiety (p=0.042). Their SUD decreased significantly as well (p=0.002), as did their ability to approach the feared stimulus (p=0.046). All of these p values were outstanding.

The same results happened if they received EFT first, or after the deep-breathing aspect. When students received EFT first, the positive effects of the tapping remained through the deep-breathing condition too.

NOTES FROM A PRACTITIONER: PHOBIAS

Case Study: Susan (Agoraphobia)

EFT practitioner Lorna Hollinger offers an account of a young mother named Susan who presented with agoraphobia. She could barely leave the house, which was having an impact on her marriage, as well as meaning she was unable to enjoy simple pleasures with her daughter, such as going to the park or the pool. Sessions were conducted via Skype for Susan, which is not uncommon when sufferers cannot leave their home.

Agoraphobia is an anxiety disorder where someone becomes afraid to leave environments they know or consider to be safe. In severe cases, a person may avoid leaving their home (the only safe environment they have) for days, months, or even years. Translated, agoraphobia means "fear of the marketplace." Public places (such as supermarkets, shopping centers, trams, trains, planes, and airports) tend to be feared the most.

In Susan's case, she told Lorna she had a voucher for a beauty salon, and she would like to go. Lorna asked Susan how high her intensity was when simply "thinking" about going out to the salon. Her SUD rating was 10+.

They tapped several rounds while Susan thought about going out. After five rounds of tapping, Susan's SUD had reduced to a 4. Lorna asked Susan to visualize herself with her keys in her hand, walking to her front door. She was asked to tell Lorna what she saw, and when her emotions peaked.

Her emotions peaked to a SUD rating of 10 again when she visualized herself near her front door. They paused and tapped, repeating "going out of the house." This took six rounds of tapping to bring her SUD down to a 2.

They repeated the visualization with Susan's SUD peaking to a 5 as she imagined herself turning the door handle. They tapped and repeated, "going out of the house" another four rounds, and this brought her SUD rating back down to a 2.

At this point Lorna asked Susan if she would feel okay to actually pick up her keys and walk to her front door. Susan agreed and tapped on her collarbone point as she walked down the corridor. She continued tapping while she opened her own front door.

They tapped for four rounds while repeating "I am safe." Susan was still feeling anxious, so they continued tapping and repeating "I am safe" until Susan indicated that she was feeling much better.

Lorna asked Susan again what her SUD rating was on "thinking" about going out. She said she was much calmer and didn't feel anxious about that at all, which she hadn't experienced in many months.

Lorna gently suggested to Susan that she could consider taking a step outside if she wanted to. And to Susan's own surprise, she did. However, as she stood on the veranda, she jingled her keys and said she felt her stomach tighten and the panic rise. Lorna talked Susan through the various *aspects* of the jingling keys to identify her trigger.

Susan was able to identify that many years prior she had been driving her car and had a panic attack while stopped at a traffic light. She had to be removed from her car, and her parents had to collect her. She had associated the jingling of the keys with this incident. This appeared to be a contributor to her panic attacks.

Lorna asked Susan to recount the incident while tapping through the points. She described how she had been following her boyfriend's car and how she was in a location that she didn't know. Her SUD peaked at 10+ at this point in telling the story.

They continued tapping and repeating "I am safe" until Susan felt better. She continued her story, including feeling stress and pressure her boyfriend put on her. Again they tapped through the points, repeating "I am safe." This statement seemed to have a significant impact for Susan.

As she remembered the incident, they tapped on "I am safe, I am no longer with him, I'm a grown woman, I have my own family, I have a husband who loves me, I am safe." They continued this for five rounds until Susan looked very calm and tired. Her SUD rating at this stage was approximately a 2 out of 10.

Lorna asked Susan how she now felt about being on her veranda, and she said she felt fine. She asked Susan if she could step onto her front path (only if she wanted to), and she did. Lorna offered to walk up to the gate with her if she wanted to (via Skype), and for Susan to let her know if there was any increasing anxiety.

Susan chose to tap on her collarbone point as she walked up her path and onto the sidewalk. She stopped tapping on her sidewalk and just stood as the widest grin came across her face. Lorna was surprised to see tears roll down Susan's cheeks, but they were tears of success and joy.

Case Study: Sandra (Needle Phobia)

EFT practitioner Margaret Munoz shared with me about working with a client on a needle phobia. This phobia is considered to affect up to 10 percent of a population. Most fear the sight, thought, or feeling of needles; and the primary symptom is fainting due to a decrease of blood pressure.

This case gives a thorough picture of how distressing phobias can be, but how effective tapping is to assist.

Margaret received an urgent phone call from Sandra, who'd been referred because of a severe needle phobia. She was pregnant and needed to have a blood test done, which was scheduled for the following day—so she was really feeling under pressure. The only way they could connect in that time frame was by telephone.

It became apparent that the phobia was indeed severe, and had been there since she was three and a half years old. Sandra had a vivid memory of herself screaming as her mother held her down while the family doctor put an injection in her bottom. She was also held down when she had her appendix out at seven years old, and mentioned difficulties when she had thyroid surgery as an adult.

Now at 38 years old, Sandra had managed to avoid needles and blood tests for a long time. She had made one attempt to have the blood taken while pregnant, and had fled. She was terrified she would "freak out" again, panic, want to run, and be crying and hysterical or faint as she had in the past.

Talking about the needle made Sandra feel sick, feel tightness in her chest, and have difficulty breathing. Margaret started with some tapping (while on the telephone) on these physical symptoms, and Sandra reported that her shoulders were less hunched, the tightness had lifted, and her breathing was easier.

Once Sandra was feeling stable, Margaret asked her to tell the story of her past experiences, but they tapped the whole time. The memory that truly bothered Sandra was the first one as a little girl, and she could even remember what the doctor was wearing and exactly what the room looked like.

After this, however, Sandra was expressing so much fear about what she thought was going to happen the following day that Margaret asked her to imagine every step of the procedure. They started by imagining walking in the door and going up to the counter and included Sandra sitting and reading a magazine in the waiting room. They tapped until she could imagine sitting there calmly and looking around the room. Margaret also included many choice statements about being safe.

Margaret and Sandra diligently worked through all of the aspects, including when the receptionist or doctor called her name, walking down the corridor, entering the room with the place where she was to sit and all the equipment, the tourniquet and the tightness of it that she so hated, the bulging of the vein, the ache in her arm, putting in the needle, feeling sick and wanting to pull the needle out and run, having the nurse say she needed another vial, and seeing any blood.

Interestingly, Sandra became aware that she was actually afraid of *letting go* of the phobia. They tapped on her resistance and the possibility that if the phobia wasn't there, then she would have to go through with the blood test, and maybe she thought that she would die. Hence the phobia—it was there to protect her from dying. So they did several rounds of tapping on the fear of dying and making more choices around being safe.

Sandra was incredibly grateful to be able to get the blood test done after the session, but even more excited when it became apparent that the phobia was totally gone, and she could now go for a blood test on her own.

Margaret received e-mails from time to time from Sandra. One said she had managed to endure a doctor who couldn't find her vein, and another one said she had just succeeded in having nine vials of blood taken!

All in all, EFT does stand out as a unique way to calm the body as a stress-management tool and address irrational fears associated with phobias. However, let's turn now to how it has been used to support physical and medical issues.

MENTAL ILLNESS: SCHIZOPHRENIA

The use of EFT for chronic mental illness is now emerging. Conditions such as schizophrenia are characterized by profound disruption in cognition and emotion, affecting the most fundamental human attributes: language, thought, perception, affect, and sense of self. Negative emotions in schizophrenia (stress, anxiety, depression, anger, guilt, despair, worry, excessive joy, great sadness, crying, and helplessness) are also common, and profoundly impact functioning.

One study in Indonesia has examined the impact of EFT for reducing the level of depression, anxiety, and stress in five patients with schizophrenia.[7]

EFT significantly improved all three negative emotions ($p<0.017$) in patients, and nurses have since been able to use the technique to reduce stress levels in patients at the psychiatric hospital.

MENTAL ILLNESS: OBSESSIVE-COMPULSIVE DISORDER

The use of EFT for other psychiatric conditions has been explored, albeit in single studies to date.

An evaluation of tapping for sufferers of obsessive-compulsive disorder (OCD) has been conducted.[8] OCD is characterized by unreasonable thoughts and fears (obsessions) that can lead to compulsive behaviors. It is an anxiety disorder and often centers on themes such as a fear of germs or the need to arrange objects in a specific manner. These recurring unwanted thoughts, images, or impulses, as well as obsessions and repetitive rituals, are typically very distressing for a sufferer.

In this study, 70 individuals with a diagnosis of OCD were assigned to a self-help tapping group or progressive muscle relaxation (PMR) group for a period of four weeks. They all completed baseline assessment over the Internet, including standard outcome measures for OCD and depression. They were then sent self-help manuals (including video demonstrations of the technique) to self-apply EFT or PMR.

From the participants' perspective, they felt the tapping was more helpful than the PMR (30 percent versus 19 percent, respectively); and 72 percent indicated they would continue to use tapping, compared with only 48 percent for PMR. However, there was no evidence for a stronger decline of OCD symptoms under tapping on any of the psychometric measures.

The authors argued the study did not support bold claims about the effectiveness of tapping as a stand-alone technique. However, it was not delivered in person, and there was no report of how often participants engaged in the technique. OCD diagnoses were not verified, and the techniques may not have been implemented correctly.

Single-case studies on the use of EFT for conditions such as OCD have been more positive, and working with someone face-to-face compared with online delivery may be vital for success.

ADDICTION

This bring us to the question of whether EFT is useful for addictions. A pilot study examining psychological symptoms in addiction treatment found using EFT to reduce stress-related symptoms might actually reduce the risk of relapse in addiction.[9]

Participants were attending a weekend workshop focused on addiction conducted by four EFT Masters. Of the 100 who attended, 39 participated, and 28 completed the 90-day follow-up. The sample was predominantly female (71.8 percent), with an average age of 54 years old (range 35 to 78 years old).

Everyone completed the SA-45 that is a short form of the Derogatis Symptom Checklist (SCL-90). It measures the severity and the breadth of symptoms and nine other areas: anxiety, depression, obsessive-compulsive behavior, phobic anxiety, hostility, interpersonal sensitivity, paranoia, psychoticism, and somatization.

Significant reductions in psychological distress occurred with improvements in the intensity and range of psychological symptoms, in addition to anxiety and obsessive-compulsive symptoms. These were all maintained at follow-up 90 days later, providing evidence for lasting therapeutic effect of EFT.

The authors acknowledged there was no comparison or control group, and the sample size was small. Practitioners also taught

EFT differently in the workshop. Some demonstrated with volunteers, others focused on addictive cravings, and another used EFT to counter the effects of adverse childhood experiences. However, as a pilot study, it at least supported the notion that EFT may be effective to consider for addiction concerns.

Smoking

I have conducted one of the only studies investigating EFT for quitting smoking. A single eight-hour smoking-cessation session using EFT was offered to employees of a large nutritional company in 2011, and was followed with a 45-minute individual session one week later.[10] Participants all voluntarily engaged in the treatment. Before beginning the intensive eight-hour session, all participants completed a survey asking about their previous successes and failures in their quit attempts; family history; emotions associated with smoking and quitting; perceived costs and negatives of changing the smoking habit; benefits and positives of continuing to smoke; perceived health beliefs about smoking consequences; issues relating to the present, past, and future that may be linked to their smoking behaviors; and personal belief in the goal of quitting.

At the completion of the eight-hour session, all participants were given an EFT treatment plan that contained common beliefs/ thoughts or situations, setup statements, and reminder phrases for future tapping processes. They then had their individual 45-minute session one week after the program finished.

The specific components of the EFT and smoking program for the eight-hour intensive included the following:

- Explaining the triggers and aspects of a smoking habit, including the craving reflex and cycle and common emotions that emerge when attempting to quit

- Exploring beliefs, present-situation emotions, past emotions, and memories relating to previous quit attempts, and future concerns related to triggering situations or events

- Psychoeducation about EFT and how to do it

- The application of EFT protocols to smoking cessation, including immediate cravings, favorite time of the day to smoke, withdrawal symptoms, thoughts and beliefs, and emotions and issues associated with the past and the future that may be maintaining smoking behavior

- The positive benefits of drinking water during the quitting process

- In vivo exposure where participants engaged in smoking cigarettes (outside) while doing the EFT process

- Aspects involved in the quitting process (e.g., psychological reversal where one part of the individual wants to change and another part, energetic or subconscious, is resistant to the change; hidden benefits in continuing to smoke; or feelings of deprivation)

- The use of positive statements and "I choose" setup statements

- Future visualizations of being a nonsmoker, and installing positive and negative beliefs attached to success

For one male (34 years) in the group program, the feeling of something in his mouth was uncovered during the EFT process. "I've tried to quit before and always ended up having three packets of soothers a day instead. I didn't realize how intense the need was to have something in my mouth."

A 40-year-old female client in the group shared at the end of the eight-hour intensive: "I have no cravings, and I'm not missing it." She reported a week later, "I was worried I'd replace it [smoking] with food, but I haven't. I still haven't missed them [the cigarettes]."

NOTES FROM A PRACTITIONER: SMOKING

Conrad was a 48-year-old married man with two adolescent sons. He worked full-time as a supervisor for the nutritional company. As part of the EFT smoking group program, he discussed wanting to quit smoking in order to be "fitter." He had previously attempted to quit 12 months earlier by going cold turkey, but had recommenced smoking as part of a celebration.

Conrad reported having smoked 30 cigarettes a day since he was 16 years old, that his sons both smoked, and that his wife used to but had quit 23 years earlier. He reported drinking alcohol in moderation (two beers a night) for relaxation purposes, and that he was mostly fit and healthy despite smoking. He did state, though, that he felt "gluggy in the chest" most mornings, which he attributed to smoking.

He listed the following reasons for why he enjoyed smoking:

- It was relaxing and part of his lifestyle.

- It calmed his nerves.

- It had a mellowing effect for him.

- It gave him a reason to have a break at work.

In the individual session that followed the group program, Conrad reported still having had a craving for cigarettes even though he had not smoked for one week, and part of him did not want to smoke. Using EFT, this craving was addressed with the statement "Even though I want this smoke [cigarette], but I don't, I accept myself anyway." Conrad rated his SUD as a 2 out of 10 after one round of tapping, and he reported that it was not quite targeting the feeling he was experiencing.

When the wording was changed to "Even though I have this habit, and I don't want to have this habit anymore, I accept myself," Conrad initially rated the statement as a 9 out of 10. Three rounds later, he rated the statement as a 1 out of 10.

Using EFT, we targeted certain feeling states Conrad reported. These included being angry that he was quitting smoking, partly worried about his health (chest feeling), and disappointed in himself as a poor role model for his sons. He also blamed himself for their smoking habits. By addressing each of these with a tapping statement, he experienced a deeper aspect of the anger feeling. He recalled a memory of being 12 years old himself, and his father yelling at him to complete a chore at home. Conrad described the anger he had toward his father at that time for being told what to do when he didn't want to comply, and not being able to do anything as a 12-year-old.

In tapping on this memory and the feelings of anger toward his father, Conrad described that the anger he was currently feeling toward quitting cigarettes was similar. He said he had always wondered why he never had liked being told what to do at work and at home, and laughed out loud as he realized the connection to the memory from when he was 12 years old.

After tapping on these issues, Conrad reported a 0 out of 10 SUD rating. In the session, we engaged in in vivo exposure by having him dry drag on a unlit cigarette for the smell and sensation, to see whether this increased his intensity or craving. It did not have any effect, and Conrad still rated his craving low, as a 1.

He said that in the tapping on the "habit statement" early in the session, he had become aware of the notion that he did not have any goals in life. Through several more rounds of tapping on this, Conrad reported that he had given up a life goal many years before to become highly skilled at karate because he believed he was unfit due to smoking. He was surprised when this surfaced through the tapping.

We used EFT to address this underlying belief ("Even though I quit karate because I thought I was unfit from smoking . . ."), and several other aspects and beliefs emerged:

- If Conrad no longer smoked, how would he be able to enjoy a break from work? (He believed that without smoking he did not have a legitimate reason to go outside away from work for 5 to 10 minutes.)

- If Conrad no longer smoked, how would he connect with his sons outside on the veranda every morning, when they had their first cigarette and coffee of the day? (Feelings of worry, inadequacy, and awkwardness surfaced.)

- If Conrad no longer smoked and pursued his old goal of karate, what if he was no longer as skilled as he used to be? (Anxiety, fear, and self-consciousness emerged in his awareness.)

Tapping was used on all of the beliefs and emotions that emerged, until Conrad reached a rating of 1 out of 10 for all of them. He reported feeing "very calm and centered" when we finished the session and did not have any craving for a cigarette. He stated that he now acknowledged the belief shift that he deserved a break at work as much as the next person, and he felt confident he could act on this without smoking.

No further sessions were arranged, as the original group program and individual session were offered through the workplace. One month later, Conrad sent an e-mail as an update. He reported that there had been a family birthday celebration, and he had lit a cigar to have as part of the merriment, but had been revolted at the taste after one drag.

He had not smoked any cigarettes and still felt calm about his decision to quit. He had not noticed a need to have any breaks at work, but still felt confident to take them without needing to smoke in order to do so.

PHYSICAL CONDITIONS: PSORIASIS

Psoriasis is thought to be an immune system problem and is a chronic skin disease. The most common symptom is a rash on the skin, but sometimes the rash involves the nails or joints. It can be very painful for a sufferer and distressing because of how it looks.

There has been one small pilot study conducted for sufferers of psoriasis.[11] The aim of this study was to see if stress reduction might improve the quality of life in sufferers of psoriasis. There were 12 sufferers, and all received a six-hour EFT workshop and were instructed to use EFT daily. Their symptoms were measured using the Skindex-29 questionnaire, and psychological distress was measured in a 45-item survey. Participants were assessed pre-intervention, post-intervention, and at one- and three-month follow-ups.

Significant improvements in the severity and range of psoriasis symptoms and psychological/emotional functioning were observed for all participants, highlighting the dual benefit of EFT (i.e., psychological and physiological symptom alleviation/improvement).

Relief often was immediate and sustained, and improved over time, and may be a useful adjunct to treatment of this condition.

PHYSICAL CONDITIONS: SLEEP

EFT has been compared to sleep hygiene education (SHE) in a group-therapy format in a geriatric population.[12] Given that half of adults aged 60 or older report difficulty initiating or sleeping through the night, this is an important area. Loss of sleep in the elderly has been tied to loss of memory, decreased concentration, and decreased functional performance in daily activities.

The 20 elderly women in this study (average age was 80) were examined and given a diagnosis of insomnia by a neuropsychiatrist, and then randomly allocated into two groups. One group received SHE, and the other a form of EFT adapted for use with insomnia (they used movement and relaxation techniques to mimic the physical elements of EFT and also simplified reminder phrases for easier recall). Everyone received eight one-hour sessions: meeting twice a week for four weeks.

All women were assessed for insomnia severity, depression, anxiety, and life satisfaction before and after treatment; and follow-ups occurred at five and nine weeks. They were also instructed to self-apply EFT via the use of a cassette tape and recorder and asked to listen and follow instructions at least once per day.

While neither intervention resulted in a significant improvement in anxiety or life satisfaction, EFT was more effective than

SHE for insomnia. It was also cost effective being delivered in a group format and highlighted the potential of EFT as an effective treatment for insomnia.

PHYSICAL CONDITIONS: RESPIRATORY ISSUES

Iranian researchers conducted a unique study on the impact of EFT on immunological factors.[13] They were very interested in war veterans who had been exposed to chemical weapons and had chronic respiratory problems and war-induced psychological and physical problems.

There were 28 male veterans aged between 43 and 58 years who had pulmonary injury by mustard gas in the Iran-Iraq War between 1980 and1988. They all had mild to moderate pulmonary problems based on Global Initiative for Chronic Obstructive Lung Disease (GOLD) criteria.

All men were randomly allocated to either EFT (14) or a wait-list control group (14). Prior to any treatment, everyone completed the General Health Questionnaire (GHQ), the St. George's respiratory questionnaires (SGRQ), and immunological testing.

The EFT group received eight sessions of EFT. In the first session, the history and applications of EFT were described. Then an educational film about other patients' previous experience was shown. Afterward, the therapists helped patients identify three common distressing problems.

These problems included respiratory symptoms such as coughing and shortness of breath, immune deficiency and recurrent infectious diseases, and psychological problems like depression and anxiety.

Setup statements were used for each of these problems, which were then targeted with tapping. Participants received eight weekly, 90-minute group sessions and were asked to do daily home practices twice a day.

Following the eight-week period, all participants returned to complete the same measures, including immunological tests.

During the EFT eight-week period, the wait-list group was asked not to participate in any new intervention or treatment. They did receive the EFT after this period.

Compared to the wait-list, EFT significantly improved the men's mental health and health-related quality of life. It also significantly decreased their somatic symptoms, anxiety/insomnia, social dysfunction, and frequency and severity of respiratory symptoms.

It resulted in an increase of lymphocyte proliferation with nonspecific mitogens concanavalin A (Con A) and phytohemagglutinin (PHA), and peripheral blood IL-17. Greater proliferation is associated with a more effective immune response. IL-17 is a proinflammatory cytokine produced by activated memory T cells and has a key role in a host's defense against microbial infections such as mycobacterium tuberculosis. It has a key role in the initiation and maintenance of inflammatory responses.

Other studies have shown that stress can affect the function and number of immune cells, production of many cytokines, and reduction of lymphocyte proliferation. Other stress-management interventions, such as mindfulness-based stress reduction, have been shown to reduce the immunosuppressive effects of stressors. But this was the first on EFT and immunity.

It showed EFT may be a noninvasive approach for improving psychological and immunological factors.

PHYSICAL CONDITIONS: FIBROMYALGIA

Fibromyalgia is a chronic-pain condition that includes widespread pain and tenderness, and often fatigue and altered sleep, as well as memory and mood issues. It is one of the most common chronic pain conditions, affecting 3 to 6 percent of the world's population. There have been two research studies conducted on the effectiveness of tapping for fibromyalgia.

In the first study, 86 women diagnosed with fibromyalgia and on sick leave for at least three months were recruited in Sweden and randomly assigned to a tapping group (43) or a wait-list group (43). For those in the treatment group, an eight-week EFT treatment program was administered via the internet.[14]

All participants completed surveys related to their health, anxiety, and depression levels; thoughts related to pain; acceptance of their pain; and general self-efficacy.

The tapping group was instructed to use EFT once a day for eight weeks. For every daily session, the EFT participants registered the severity of the treated problem or symptom on the distress rating scale (1 to 10, where 1: no problem, 10: severe problem). Once a week they e-mailed their EFT distress-rating sheets to the study leader, who also instructed the participants via e-mail when needed. Those who did not e-mail any sheets were reminded with telephone calls.

Significant reductions in pain, catastrophizing thoughts (rumination, magnification, and helplessness), anxiety, and depression symptoms were observed in those who engaged in the EFT treatment. The self-reported pain decreased in the tapping group from 7 to 5; in the wait-list group, however, there was no decrease at all.

There was a high dropout rate (40 percent) for the EFT group, but about half of the dropouts did not discontinue EFT training because of a lack of effect; they did not even start the training. Therefore, while the positive results for the treatment group have to be interpreted with caution, it was a landmark study.

In another study, a student focused an entire dissertation thesis on the effectiveness of EFT on the somatic symptoms of fibromyalgia.[15] In a sample of six women diagnosed with fibromyalgia, the researchers conducted EFT in a clinical setting for half of the women (the other half were wait-listed). The average age of all women was 54.67 years, and the average number of years for being diagnosed was 12.68.

Based on self-report, all participants positively responded to a history of emotional trauma: five women reported emotional abuse, physical abuse, sexual abuse, and the sudden death of a loved one; and one reported a history of emotional abuse alone.

The investigators conducted three sequences of EFT in each of four treatment sessions. The data suggested there was improvement in overall pain (tender points) for the women; however, there was not enough information to result in statistical outcome. The decreases in pain were not statistically different from the control group, who received no treatment. However, the author argued the overall improvement in the tender-point pain in those who used EFT, and the data from within-treatment sessions, showed the great decreases in tender-point pain from sequence to sequence. Therefore, clinically it was impactful for sufferers, and future studies with larger sample sizes may confirm this.

PHYSICAL CONDITIONS: BREAST CANCER

A common reason women with breast cancer discontinue hormonal therapies is the adverse effects associated with tamoxifen and aromatase inhibitor. Aromatase inhibitors stop the production of estrogen in postmenopausal women, which turns the hormone androgen into small amounts of estrogen in the body. This means that less estrogen is available to stimulate the growth of hormone-receptor-positive breast cancer cells.

Because poor medical treatment compliance is associated with an increased risk of mortality and early recurrence of the breast cancer, one study aimed to improve the mood state, menopausal symptoms, fatigue, and pain in women with breast cancer who were receiving hormonal therapies.[16]

Self-report questionnaires were used to assess mood, pain, fatigue, endocrine (menopausal) symptoms, and hot flashes and night sweats in 41 women. They also completed a hot-flash diary at the start of the EFT program and at 6- and 12-week follow-ups. Everyone completed a seven-day home practice sheet for the first six weeks and a feedback form at six weeks, and they all were invited to attend a follow-up focus group at eight weeks.

The women received one session of EFT (three hours per week) over three weeks. Over the next nine weeks, they were asked to self-apply the technique when required.

There were statistically significant improvements at both 6 and 12 weeks in Total Mood Disturbance (anxiety, depression, and fatigue), compared to baseline.

In addition, the average fatigue interference and global scores, numbers of hot flashes, and the hot flash–problem rating score decreased at 6 and/or 12 weeks.

The findings suggested that EFT may be an effective self-help tool for women with breast cancer experiencing side effects from hormonal therapies. As a result they may be less likely to discontinue hormonal treatment.

PHYSICAL CONDITIONS: DIABETES

The prevalence of type 2 diabetes in Iran has accelerated in recent years, and more than one percent of Iranians over age 20 are affected by it each year. Researchers wanted to improve glycemic control in diabetic patients, reducing the need for costly medical services, and enhance their mental health.[17]

Because stress can result in excess glucose being released in the body for supplying energy, and diabetes being a metabolic condition where the body is not able to make full use of this excess sugar, EFT may be a way to reduce stress in the body. This may then result in diabetes sufferers being able to better control their blood-sugar levels.

In 2012, 30 patients with type 2 diabetes admitted to a Tehran hospital on full insulin doses were randomly classified into two groups: an EFT group and a control group.

The sample included 27 female and 3 male diabetic patients ranging from 40 to 65 years. Blood glucose testing (glycosylated hemoglobin testing, HbA1C) was used, and EFT participants received 12 sessions of treatment.

Results showed that EFT was effective in controlling blood glucose levels in diabetic patients and was proposed as a way to assist other physical, metabolic, and glandular disorders.

PHYSICAL CONDITIONS: BRAIN INJURY

It has been suggested that the "invisible wounds" of returning war soldiers include post-traumatic stress disorder, major depression, and traumatic brain injury (TBI). TBI has been called the "signature injury" of military personnel deployed to the war zones of Afghanistan and Iraq.

TBI ranges from being mild (an external injury to the brain with confusion, disorientation, or a loss or altered state of consciousness for 30 minutes or less) to moderate (involving a loss of consciousness and post-traumatic amnesia) to severe.

Because studies of EFT for PTSD have been positive, Dr. Church and colleagues sought to assess whether the resolution of PTSD symptoms using EFT would also correlate with a reduction in TBI symptoms.

A group of 59 veterans (aged 24 to 86 years, average of 52 years) with clinical levels of post-traumatic stress disorder symptoms were randomized into either an EFT group (30) or standard-care wait-list control (29).[18] All participants had to be under the care of a clinician from a Veterans Affairs or other licensed health-care facility. The EFT intervention was delivered as a complementary and supporting supplement to their standard care.

The participants completed assessments at the start of treatment, after three EFT sessions, after six EFT sessions, at treatment completion, and at three- and six-month follow-ups. The measures included demographic characteristics; somatoform disorders; pain; lifestyle choices; alcohol, cigarette, recreational drug, and prescription drug use; and TBI symptoms.

EFT was introduced to participants as peer-to-peer coaching rather than as therapy. Six hour-long sessions of EFT were delivered individually by 15 EFT-certified coaches either in the coach's office or by telephone. During each session, coaches and participants created lists of traumatic events and then self-rated their level of emotional distress (ranging from 0: no distress to 10: highest distress possible).

Participants self-applied EFT and worked through each of the traumatic memories with the coach. Participants were encouraged to keep tapping in between sessions as well.

One participant in the EFT group dropped out after three sessions, and four subjects in the control group dropped out before the second session. There were 29 in the EFT group and 20 in the standard-care wait-list group who completed assessments and all six EFT sessions.

At the three-month follow-up, data were obtained for 25 in the EFT group and 17 in the standard-care wait-list group; at six months, the numbers were 26 and 13, respectively. Those subjects lost to attrition cited an uncomfortable level of emotion during memory recall, the burden of filling out forms, and a lack of time as their reasons for not completing the study.

A significant percentage of veterans dropped below the clinical threshold for PTSD after six sessions of EFT (86 percent, $p <$ .0001) and remained subclinical at three-month and six-month follow-ups.

Compared with the start of treatment, significant reductions in TBI symptoms were found after only three sessions, with a further reduction after six months (of 41 percent, $p <$ .0021). Participant gains were maintained on three-month and six-month follow-ups ($p <$ .0006).

This study highlighted the potential for partial TBI rehabilitation after successful PTSD treatment, and the possibility of EFT being integral to this.

PHYSICAL CONDITIONS: CHRONIC PAIN

The first study to look at EFT for chronic-pain reduction in adults was led by Nick Ortner.[19] Fifty adults with chronic pain (minimum three months) participated in a three-day workshop.

Their pain was measured on the Pain Catastrophizing Scale and the Multidimensional Pain Inventory immediately before and after treatment, and at the one-month and six-month follow-ups.

The majority of the group were women (86 percent), and the average age was 57 years (a range of 35 to 72 years). When asked to rate their pain on a scale of 0 to 10 (0: no pain, 10: maximum), the average rating was 8, indicating severe pain.

At the workshop EFT was demonstrated to the group over three eight-hour days, but they self-applied it. They were able to volunteer in a demonstration in front of the group if they chose. Trained volunteers were also available for individual tapping sessions if needed. Everyone was encouraged to continue using EFT after the workshop (although data was not collected on whether they did).

Participants were also able to arrange three phone calls with Nick Ortner for additional tapping sessions, which would then be recorded for them. Few participants utilized this option, but all participants received two audio meditative tapping sessions (approximately seven minutes long) for their individual use.

Significant reductions were found on each of the Pain Catastrophizing Scale items (rumination, magnification, and helplessness) and the total score (decreases of 43 percent, $p < .001$).

On the Multidimensional Pain Inventory, significant improvements were observed in pain severity, interference, life control, affective distress, and dysfunctional composite ($p < .001$).

Nine subjects did not complete the measures at the one-month follow-up, leaving 41 subjects. Between one month and six months, an additional 7 subjects were lost to follow-up, leaving 34 subjects for analysis.

However, participants available maintained their significant improvements in Pain Catastrophizing Scale scores at the one-month and six-month follow-ups, with the exception of magnification at one-month follow-up. At the six-month follow-up, reductions were still maintained on this scale (decrease of 42 percent, $p < .001$), but only on the life-control item for the Multidimensional Pain Inventory.

EFT definitely reduced pain severity as an immediate strategy, and also improved participants' ability to live with their pain. The group continued to report an improved sense of control and ability to cope with their chronic pain over time, and EFT was considered a useful tool in the self-management of pain.

In 2016, I too explored the effectiveness of EFT for chronic pain in a local persistent-pain program that includes EFT as part of its approach.[20]

We initially looked at the impact, challenges, and current experience of chronic-pain sufferers in an anonymous, online, open-ended survey. This aspect of the study highlighted the issues sufferers had with employment, interpersonal relationships, and emotions. An overwhelming 82 percent discussed the stigma they experienced from health professionals who didn't believe the extent of their pain, and only 4 percent indicated they received any pain relief from psychological treatment.

This snapshot seems to be the norm for sufferers, rather than the exception, and we took this information and designed a brief four-hour EFT group session. This was delivered on a single day as part of a local 12-month pain program for sufferers.

Most of the 24 people in the group were women (84 percent), over 50 years of age (72 percent), and married (44 percent). It is important to note they didn't choose to be involved—everyone in the pain program at that time was included.

An overview of tapping was provided at the beginning of the session, and the whole group engaged in tapping exercises for two hours with the facilitator. After this they formed small groups of six (with an EFT practitioner in each as a support person and guide) in order to engage in more specific tapping statements.

They focused on more personal experiences of pain (e.g., one participant tapped on pain related to a motor vehicle accident, and another tapped on sciatic pain which resulted from the position of their baby during pregnancy).

Over the four hours, sufferers reported a significant decrease in the severity (decrease of 12.04 percent, $p=0.044$) and impact (decrease of 17.62 percent, $p=0.008$) of their pain. Their overall psychological distress improved by 36.67 percent (p < 0.001), and their depression scores improved by 29.86 percent (p=0.007). They also reported a decrease in anxiety (by 41.69 percent, p < 0.001) and stress (by 38.48 percent, p=0.001). You can see these significance levels are excellent.

Only half the sample indicated they were still using it at the six-month follow-up, but a main effect of time was still significant. This means there was a difference in symptoms between the start of the program and six months later. But when we drilled down, we didn't find any significant results at the individual time points. This can happen when the sample size is small. We also lacked a comparison group, and a longer follow-up period may have been beneficial. These are all things to keep in mind moving forward.

PHYSICAL CONDITIONS: SHOULDER ISSUES

Dr. Church has conducted several studies on shoulder issues.[21] In 2008, he investigated psychological symptoms and range of movement in 47 individuals with clinically verified shoulder joint impairments. The focus was on whether the treatment of emotional trauma had an effect on physiological function. Psychological conditions such as anxiety and depression were measured using a 45-item self-assessment survey, and pain was measured on a 10-point Likert-type scale.

Everyone received a single 30-minute intervention after being randomized into either an EFT group (16 subjects) or a diaphragmatic-breathing group (18 subjects). There were also 13 people who were a no-treatment baseline control group.

Greater improvements in pain were seen in the EFT group both immediately following treatment and at follow-up 30 days after treatment. At follow-up, range of movement continued to improve for both treatment groups; however, greater improvements were seen in those who received EFT.

More recently Dr. Church has looked at frozen shoulder syndrome and the effects of EFT.[22] The study included 37 participants with frozen shoulder consisting of limited range of motion (ROM) and pain. They were randomized into a wait-list or one of two treatment groups (EFT or diaphragmatic breathing).

Everyone completed questionnaires on ROM, their pain levels, and the breadth and depth of psychological conditions such as anxiety and depression before and after a 30-minute treatment session, and 30 days later.

One treatment group received EFT, while the other received an identical cognitive/exposure protocol but with diaphragmatic breathing (DB) substituted for the tapping stimulation. No significant improvement in any psychological symptom was found in the wait-list.

Participants in both the EFT and DB groups demonstrated significant improvement in psychological symptoms and pain after their session. The follow-up showed that both groups maintained their gains for pain; however, EFT was superior to DB.

Only the EFT group maintained their gains for psychological symptoms, however ($p < 0.001$). Large EFT treatment effects were found, with a Cohen's d=0.9 for anxiety and pain, and d=1.1 for depression.

The ROM was not significantly improved, although the EFT group showed a greater trend for enhanced ROM. Future research should seek to have larger sample sizes to ascertain if this would respond. What was interesting, though, was that reductions in psychological distress were also associated with reduced pain as well as with improved ROM. This may point to the relationship between emotional issues and physical pain/distress.

NOTES FROM A PRACTITIONER: PHYSICAL PAIN

EFT practitioner Johann Gray demonstrates in this case that EFT doesn't always have to be serious for chronic issues, even though serious issues such as resistance and inertia are being addressed.

Mel's left knee had been bothering her for six months. It was a gradual thing, and she did not know when she originally injured it. She could remember it hurting a lot when she put her ski boots on, and her husband had to help her get in and out of the boots. That was six months ago. But now the pain was excruciating, and she could barely get her underwear on. Her SUD rating was 8 out of 10 when bending the knee.

Johann asked Mel what was going on in her life six months ago. She talked about managing colleagues who complained about everything and had very negative attitudes. Mel did not like having confronting conversations that would "rock the boat," so she would often work overtime to fix things instead of asking the right person to take responsibility. Then she felt terrible about being a bad mother to her children, as she was only meant to be working part-time. She was working all the time, even when she was at home.

Mel thought that her knee could be sore because she was overweight. She also had an internal belief or rule she followed: that overweight people should not exercise, as it was "gross."

Johann and Mel were laughing hysterically as she tapped about her pain when she put on her underwear; the awkward situations that she found herself in at work, taking on too much herself and never asking for help; and her longing to be more active with her kids, at the same time judging how obscene she must look while moving vigorously in her exercise clothes.

After a number of rounds, Johann asked Mel what was coming up for her. She said that she would like to see a physiotherapist, but she felt a lot of resistance to making the phone call. She had the same issue with her overdue Pap smear and getting her hair colored. Just the thought of making the phone calls to book the appointments was overwhelming. Mel said it was because she wasn't sure if she could keep the appointments.

She would prefer to show up whenever she had the free time instead of making an appointment in advance, as she had no idea what emergency would come up each day, and she was simply terrified of making personal commitments.

They did several rounds of tapping in peals of laughter about how challenging it was to use her smartphone to dial her physiotherapist, and about telling the receptionist that she would not be able to commit, because the future was way too unpredictable.

Then Mel had another revelation. She said she did not want to "hear the news." She did not want to be told what was wrong with her and what she needed to do about it. She thought it was better to be in a vague place where she could guess what her health issues might be, and not do anything specifically about them because it wasn't official.

At the end of the session, Mel's SUD rating remained at 8 out of 10. However, Mel said she would call the physiotherapist to make an appointment, and Johann considered that to be a successful conclusion, as EFT had led the client to a clear course of action. Johann explained to Mel that perhaps her knee pain was a metaphor for something in her life: something she would rather put up with because she did not want to be told what was wrong and what she had to do.

Mel had a follow-up session because she had seen her physiotherapist several times, but she was refusing to do the exercises he had prescribed. The physiotherapist told Mel that if she did the exercises, her knee would be fine in six weeks. Johann and Mel laughed about how she had put up with the pain for six months, when it would only take six weeks to fix. And now that she had made the effort to see the physiotherapist, Mel was at a loss as to why she had no motivation to do the exercises. Her SUD rating was 10 out of 10 in terms of resistance to the exercises.

Johann asked Mel to just tap on her collarbone point while they talked. They laughed as Mel said she had only done the exercises once, and it was at the physiotherapist's office when he was teaching them to her. She said the exercises were easy to do, but she just didn't have time for them.

Johann asked Mel to do the exercises in front of her so that they could time how long they took. Mel said she couldn't, that was the problem. She needed to find her yoga mat, and she thought it might be in the attic. This was the worst place it could be, because her knee would make it hard for her to climb up the ladder.

After doing a tapping round about her frustration with her yoga mat being out of reach in the attic, Mel had an *aha!* moment that she could ask her husband to get it for her. At this point, her husband knocked on the door. They laughed at the timeliness of his appearance.

"Here he is," Mel said. "Do you think you could look in the attic for my yoga mat?"

And her husband replied, "Your yoga mat? It's not in the attic. I saw it down here." Her husband instantly gave her the yoga mat.

They laughed so hard about how long she agonized about it, and how easily it was resolved after she asked for help.

Mel did her exercises, and she and Johann could hardly stop laughing as most of the exercises were actually done off the yoga mat and in total only took two minutes. They did a few rounds about her rule that overweight people "should not exercise as they look ridiculous." Mel realized that not doing her exercises was more ridiculous than anything else, as she did not even have to change her outfit to do them. Her SUD rating went down to 0 as her resistance completely dissolved.

· ·

Several months later, Mel's knee was better, and she laughed again when she said, "I can't even remember which knee it was." Aside from the knee, Mel happily gave examples of initiating some difficult conversations at work. These cleared the air and improved her life altogether. "I never would have done that before!" she said.

PHYSICAL CONDITIONS: EYESIGHT

You may be wondering, *How EFT could possibly work for eyesight issues?* Consider this statement: "He/she made me so mad I couldn't see straight!"

Studies have shown that anger can actually redden the eyes and swell the minor blood vessels. Rage can also cause vision to blur and "warp" so that the person actually "can't see straight" when they are too angry. Emotions like this became the focus of Carol's study.

Participants already familiar with EFT chose to participate in an eight-week EFT study focused on eyesight concerns. There were 120 who completed the program, and 82 percent were women. Most participants (nearly 70 percent) had not had their eyesight tested during the three months prior to the study; however, 80 percent indicated that they wore glasses for vision correction. The average age was 52, with just over half the participants in their 50s.

Each study participant was sent weekly e-mails with a topic related to eyesight (e.g., fear, anger, guilt, hurt). Three full sets of EFT setup statements were provided. Each set had one tapping round focusing on the problem, followed by a second round that focused on the possibility of a solution.

Everyone was asked to use EFT once a day, and 86 percent reported that they tapped seven or more times by the end of week one. At the end of the second week, the number of people tapping seven or more times dropped slightly to about 82 percent. For the next three weeks, this trend held fairly well. During the last three weeks, the number of people who reported tapping seven or more times decreased again to mid-to-lower 70 percent range. However, most people appeared to comply well with the instructions.

There was a significant difference between men and women in terms of overall eyesight improvement (p=.022), in that women's eyesight improved more than men's. Nearly 75 percent of participants indicated that an improvement occurred in their vision during and by the end of the study, and 50 percent indicated that their nearsightedness improved. Over 42 percent of the participants who reported being farsighted indicated an improvement.

Participants were asked, "Which emotion you tapped on caused the most dramatic changes in your eyesight?" Anger was mentioned 42 times, far more often than any other emotion.

While more than 28 percent reported that they sought additional EFT help, there was no significant difference between those who did this and those who did not in terms of their overall eyesight improvement.

Curiously, there were no statistically significant differences in age groups in terms of overall improvement in eyesight. This is interesting considering the popular belief that eyesight deterioration coincides with the aging process. While it was never published, the actual study complete with instructions is available through the Vitality Living College website.[23]

While this study did have its limitations (e.g., there was no comparison or control treatment, participants were not monitored throughout the study, and there was no formal eye testing), it was an interesting study and one worth reproducing.

TAKE-HOME POINTS

As is becoming clear, EFT has had a remarkable amount of research conducted, and in many areas.

I'd like to end this chapter with an e-mail I received from someone who attended one of my trainings. After I shared about the curious outcomes of Carol Look's unpublished pilot study on EFT for eyesight issues, one person decided to self-apply the program as per Carol's protocol. Three months after my workshop, I received the following e-mail:

> *Hi Peta,*
> *You may recall November last year when I did your tapping course on the Gold Coast, I was interested in Carol Look's tapping guide for my eyes.*
> *I tapped extensively on all the emotions I could think of at*

the time (in accordance with her guidelines) and went to my optometrist for an eye test earlier this year. I felt like my eyes had changed, because my glasses seemed blurry at certain distances. I had always had astigmatism (diagnosed in my 20s) and in later years have had a graduated lens for reading.

Anyway, my optometrist checked my eyes and told me nothing had changed. I told him about the tapping, but all he did was check my eyes from the base point on my script. I have been battling on throughout the year and made do with my glasses.

Times are tough, though, and I was thinking of discontinuing my private health insurance, so thought that I would have another test and get another set of glasses before I did that.

Anyway, I had an exam yesterday, and the results were interesting! I went to a different optometrist and told her that I wanted her to check my eyes from scratch and tell me what was wrong with them and that she couldn't look at my glasses until she completed the test!

Interestingly, as she was checking my eyes, she never mentioned astigmatism; and I think she was a little surprised when she discovered that my glasses were prescribed for this. Anyway, she told me that my eyes were not too bad! I will see how the new glasses go!!! I believe that I am slightly shortsighted and slightly longsighted. I will have to tap on that!!!

Kind Regards,
Debbie

Perhaps this area, like many, is worth investigating further.

OTHER TAPPING TECHNIQUES

While the main body of empirical research in the last few decades has focused on EFT, other tapping approaches do exist. Several of these have been tested for effectiveness in various types of trials, and these are explored in this chapter.

THOUGHT FIELD THERAPY

As mentioned in Chapter 2, Dr. Roger Callahan founded Thought Field Therapy (TFT) after using specific sequences of acupoints for different emotional problems. These are termed "algorithms."

In 2016, TFT was declared an effective evidence-based therapy for reducing trauma and stressor-related disorders by the National Registry of Evidence-Based Programs and Practices (NREPP) of the Substance Abuse and Mental Health Services Administration (SAMHSA).[1] According to the NREPP, TFT can be considered an effective therapy, which would then warrant further study. This was indeed a landmark in the field of energy psychology and tapping techniques.

There has been a range of studies conducted on TFT.

PTSD

An initial study in 2002 of 31 clients (aged 5 to 48 years) who received TFT examined its impact on trauma symptoms after 30 days.[2] Pretest and posttest total scores showed a significant drop in all symptom subgroupings of the criteria for PTSD.

Many other studies have focused on the effectiveness of TFT with genocide survivors. Fifty orphaned adolescents who had been suffering with symptoms of PTSD since the Rwandan genocide 12 years earlier received a single TFT session.[3] Their symptoms significantly decreased (p < .0001), and informal interviews with the adolescents and the caregivers indicated dramatic reductions of PTSD symptoms such as flashbacks, nightmares, bed-wetting, depression, isolation, difficulty concentrating, jumpiness, and aggression.

Following the study, the self and peer use of TFT became part of the culture at the orphanage; and at one-year follow-up, the initial improvements had been maintained.

Another study of the efficacy of TFT in reducing PTSD symptoms involved 145 adult survivors of the 1994 genocide in Rwanda and randomly assigned participants to a TFT treatment or a wait-list control group.[4] Reduced trauma symptoms for the group receiving TFT were found for all measures, and trauma-symptom reductions were sustained at a two-year follow-up assessment.

Community-Led Studies on Trauma

Because TFT is a self-help treatment, it is considered to be easy to disseminate through the development of community-based partnerships of trained mental-health practitioners and trained community leaders.

One study examined the use of TFT after a large-scale traumatic event.[5] TFT techniques were originally taught to Rwandan community leaders, who then provided one-time, individual, trauma-focused TFT interventions to 164 adult survivors of the 1994 Rwandan genocide in their native language, Kinyarwanda. They ranged in age from 18 to 100 years (average was 47.7 years), and the majority were female (141 people, 86 percent; male 23 people, 14 percent).

Eighty-three (50.6 percent) participants reported that they had previously sought treatment for their problems since the genocide of 1994. All participants also met diagnostic criterion for PTSD.

The Trauma Symptom Inventory (TSI) and the Modified Post-traumatic Stress Disorder Symptom Scale (MPSS) translated into Kinyarwanda were used. There were 36 Rwandan therapists who were respected community leaders from the Byumba and Kigali regions of Rwanda and all spoke the native language, Kinyarwanda. The therapists also spoke French and/or English.

After participants agreed to the study, they were randomly allocated to an active TFT group or a wait-list control group. The wait-list did receive the TFT treatment as well, but not until after the active treatment was complete.

The therapists were contacted one year after the study completion. They reported they treated an average of 37.50 people and met with each client an average of 3.19 times. They had treated between 3 and 123 people, and they had seen each client between one and six times.

Despite randomization of the study, some of the pretest scores were significantly different between the treatment and control groups. These differences were found in trauma symptoms and level of PTSD symptom severity and frequency between the treatment and the wait-list control groups.

The posttest scores showed significant decreases in trauma symptoms for the treatment group on all TSI subscales and significant decreases on the MPSS frequency and severity scales.

Participants in the wait-list group also experienced significant reductions in trauma symptoms following their subsequent TFT treatment, which took place after the first posttest.

Large effect sizes (from .8 to 1.33) were found between treatment and no-treatment control conditions on the TSI subscales of Anxious Arousal, Depression, Anger/Irritability, Intrusive Experiences, Defensive Avoidance, Impaired Self-Reference, and Dissociation, as well as the MPSS frequency and severity scales.

High medium (above .60) effect sizes were found for the Tension Reduction Behavior subscale. Small effect sizes (.2) were found for the Sexual Concerns and Dysfunctional Sexual Behavior subscales. The effect size on the MPSS Frequency Scale was 1.33 on the Severity Scale, and 1.2 on the Frequency Scale.

These were generally all very strong, demonstrating the magnitude of change after the TFT treatment. While the outcomes may not be generalizable to all Rwandans or other war survivors, these initial positive outcomes suggest that a one-time, community leader–facilitated, trauma-focused TFT intervention may be beneficial with protracted PTSD in genocide survivors.

TFT treatment in a rural population in Uganda has also been delivered by 36 local community workers after receiving a two-day training.[6] They then treated 256 volunteers with symptoms suggestive of PTSD who were randomly allocated to a treatment or wait-list (control) group.

A week after treatment, the TFT group scores had improved significantly, from 58 to 26.1 based on the Posttraumatic Checklist for Civilians (PCL-C), in which scores range from 17 (no trauma) to 85 (severe PTSD). The wait-list group scores did improve without treatment, from 61.2 to 47; however, it was significantly less than the treatment group. After they received the TFT, they improved to 26.4. There was some evidence of persisting benefit 19 months later.

A Meta-analysis for Trauma

In 2017 a meta-analysis explored if participants would have a greater reduction in PTSD-specific trauma symptoms guided by TFT-trained professionals or paraprofessionals than those receiving no treatment.[7] Five studies met the qualifications for inclusion; they were conducted between 2001 and 2016. The authors searched 39 databases and also sent requests to colleagues to share any studies that had not been published.

The overall effect size for the pre- to post-TFT treatment conditions was extremely large and statistically significant (-2.27).

While the authors concluded TFT was highly effective in reducing trauma symptoms in a variety of populations and settings, they did acknowledge limitations of the review. The methodologies of the studies included were different from each other, and not every study was included. Because of the small number of experienced and approved TFT trainers, and limited funding available for large-scale randomized controlled studies, the quality of studies published may be compromised. Future reviews should address this.

Public Speaking

The application of TFT for public-speaking anxiety has also resulted in positive outcomes.[8] Single 60-minute TFT sessions were conducted with 48 people suffering public-speaking anxiety by 11 licensed and trained psychotherapists. Participants were randomly assigned to TFT or a delayed-treatment (wait-list) group.

There were 38 female and 10 male participants, ranging in age from 29 to 63 years. Everyone completed the Speaker Anxiety Scale, and they were then given a list of possible speech topics. They all chose a topic and were given three minutes to prepare a speech.

Everyone then gave the speech for three minutes, which was videotaped, in front of a live audience that was composed of other study subjects and additional persons recruited as audience members. Audience members were instructed not to respond in any way during a participant's presentation.

Following the speeches, everyone then completed the Speaker Anxiety Scale a second time. Subjects in the treatment group then received 60 minutes of TFT, after which they gave a second speech. Following the second speech, they completed the Speaker Anxiety Scale for the third and final time.

Those in the wait-list control group did not receive psychotherapy or other intervention after completing the questionnaire the first time. Four weeks later, each of them gave a second speech and filled out the measure for the third time. They then received TFT, gave a third speech, and completed the form a fourth time.

Participants in the control group showed no improvement while on the wait-list. But after both groups had received TFT, they all showed decreases in public-speaking anxiety and increases in positive measures related to anticipation of future public-speaking experiences. The effect-size reduction in anxiety for the treatment group was 1.52 (this is very high), indicating TFT did have a positive effect.

Five months after the last speech, the lead author conducted an informal follow-up with 31 (64 percent) of the treatment subjects. Of these, three reported no improvement from treatment. Twenty-five said they felt "less" apprehension in public-speaking situations and reported: "I can say what I'm thinking," and "I'm not dreading it when I have to give a presentation."

These interviews may have biases toward the level of positive reports because of demand characteristics. This refers to subtle cues that can make a participant aware of what the experimenter expects to find, and therefore how participants are expected to behave. They may then match this. Further research in this area is warranted.

Anxiety Disorders

TFT has also been explored for a wide range of anxiety disorders. In a study of 45 patients who were randomly allocated to a treatment (23) or wait-list (22), the TFT group had a significantly better outcome on two measures of anxiety and one measure of function.[9] All patients were followed up one to two weeks after their TFT treatment, and at 3 and 12 months. The wait-list group did receive the TFT at the end of the study period (after 10 weeks). The significant improvement after TFT was maintained at the 3- and 12-month assessments.

- *Agoraphobia:* A 2017 study comparing the efficacy of TFT and CBT for patients with agoraphobia has been the first to do so.[10] Agoraphobia is an anxiety disorder that often develops after one or more panic attacks. Symptoms include fear and avoidance of places and situations that might cause feelings of panic, entrapment, helplessness, or embarrassment (e.g., public transport, shopping malls).

  Seventy-two adult patients who met the diagnostic criteria for either "panic disorder with agoraphobia" or "agoraphobia without a history of panic disorder" were randomly assigned to a CBT treatment (24) or TFT (24) or a three-month wait-list (24). After the waiting period, those patients were again randomly assigned to either CBT (12) or TFT (12). Seventy-one of the patients had panic disorder with agoraphobia, while one patient had agoraphobia without panic disorder.

  Everyone completed the Anxiety and Related Disorders Interview Schedule with an interviewer and the following self-report measures: the Mobility Inventory for Agoraphobia (or assessing severity of agoraphobic avoidance behavior), the Beck Depression Inventory, the Beck Anxiety Inventory, the Agoraphobic Cognitions Questionnaire, and the Body Sensations Questionnaire.

  The TFT intervention included five 50-to-55-minute sessions of individual therapy, and the CBT intervention included 12 sessions of 50 to 55 minutes each.

Both CBT and TFT showed better results than the wait-list control group (p < 0.001) at posttreatment. However, there were no differences between the CBT and TFT groups after treatment and at 12-month follow-up (p=0.33 and p=0.90, respectively).

However, at the 12-month follow-up, 18 (50 percent) of the CBT patients and 10 (28 percent) of the TFT patients no longer met the diagnostic criteria for agoraphobia (p=0.09).

This was a rigorous study; and even though TFT wasn't superior to CBT, what this shows is it was comparable. Further studies may strengthen the argument that TFT is not just promising, but effective for anxiety disorders.

- *Blood-injection-injury phobia (needle phobia):* A study of needle phobia examined whether TFT could reduce or eliminate phobic symptomology.[11] There were 21 participants aged 11 to 50 years (average 37 years), and 14 were female, seven were male. The length of suffering the phobia ranged up to 16 years. Of the group, eight people knew family members who also suffered the same phobia. There were 19 people who had never had any treatment at all, and the remaining two had tried hypnosis and psychotherapy.

  What was important to note was that many of these participants were in need of medical treatment; but because of their phobia, they were unable to commence this. For example, one woman had been diagnosed with cancer and had not commenced her chemotherapy program because of her intense fear. Another wanted to have a child but wouldn't allow herself to because of the potential procedures during the pregnancy that involved needles.

  Everyone completed the Fear Survey Schedule and then received an individual one-hour session of TFT. A hypodermic syringe was used as a test of phobic response, and the researchers observed participants' ability to look at or touch it using the Clinical Global Impressions scale.

They then waited for one month, and during this time were asked not to engage in any other treatment. Then they were reassessed with the Fear Survey Schedule and the presentation of the hypodermic syringe.

There was a significant difference pre- and post-treatment with the Fear Survey Schedule (p=0.001) but no difference between genders. There was also a significant difference in participants being able to watch others being injected (p=0.002). However, there was no significant difference for participants when exposed to the hypodermic syringe.

While findings suggested that TFT might indeed be an effective method of treating needle phobias, it was a small sample, and only used one survey instrument. In addition, longer follow-up periods are necessary to determine the true effectiveness of treatments, and larger trials are warranted.

• *Acrophobia:* An early 1997 investigation of TFT for acrophobia or fear of heights demonstrated positive outcomes in 49 college students.[12] Everyone completed the Cohen acrophobia questionnaire and also approached a four-foot ladder with the intent to climb it. They used a 0 to 10 SUD scale for their distress at each floor segment and rung, and were able to discontinue the task at any time.

All students then met with another experimenter in a separate room, and a SUD rating was obtained while they thought about an anxiety-provoking situation related to height. They were then randomly assigned to one of two groups: TFT or placebo treatment (which tapped on body parts not employed in TFT).

If the student did not obtain a rating of 0 after one round, the process (experimental or placebo control) was administered once again. Posttesting was invariably conducted after the second round. Everyone then engaged in the same SUD rating as they approached and possibly climbed the ladder.

There was a statistically significant difference between those students who received TFT and those who received the placebo tapping, with the TFT subjects showing significantly more improvement. When all the SUD ratings were averaged for each subject, the difference was more pronounced when examining the scores while the students climbed the ladder.

Unfortunately, this study has never been published in an academic journal. It has merits and stands as a useful pilot worth replicating with a comparison treatment.

- *Tinnitus:* Two case discussions of individuals suffering from psychological symptoms caused by tinnitus have been published.[13] Tinnitus is any sound that you hear in your head that is not audible externally or caused by an external source. People report different types of sounds, but it is frequently described as ear ringing, clicking, buzzing, crickets, or roaring sounds. It may be linked to exposure to loud noise, hearing loss, ear or head injuries, some diseases of the ear, ear infections, or emotional stress. It can also be a side effect of medication or a combination of all of these things without a known reason. Above all, it can be very distressing for sufferers as it impacts their quality of life and aspects such as sleeping. The aim of the TFT treatment wasn't to eradicate tinnitus, but instead to target any psychological reactions resulting from it.

  The first patient in this article, a 56-year-old married man and successful painting and sheet-rock contractor, was referred 21 weeks after a car accident. The patient was suffering anxiety and depression, although all physical injuries had healed. He reported tinnitus that had caused insomnia.

The practitioner who used TFT first treated the patient's rage at the man who had caused the car accident. He rated this as a 7 on a 0 to 10 scale. To the patient's surprise, after using TFT on this feeling, his feelings of rage were gone; and he subsequently verbalized, "Staying angry is not doing me any good. It is just making things worse."

Subsequent sessions focused on the patient's feelings of frustration about having "mental problems" and annoyance at the ringing in his ears. A follow-up session 37 days later revealed the patient's depression had subsided, as had his self-criticism and criticism of others. This also resulted in an increase of concentration, assertion, and mental energy. The patient indicated his tinnitus remained, but he was accepting of this.

The second patient was a 46-year-old married man and yacht salesman who was referred by his family physician for his insomnia, depression, and anxiety. He suffered tinnitus that would keep him awake, and the use of Valium made him feel sluggish and depressed.

The patient also described extreme anxiety regarding an upcoming yacht convention, which was the largest in his geographical region. This was because he was expected to make a number of sales and speeches about the yachts' features.

TFT focused on his anxiousness that he wouldn't sleep before the event and his worry about "Valium dependency." At the next session 27 days later, the patient reported no longer taking Valium or being upset upon awakening, generally going back to sleep within 30 minutes. He reported his speeches and sales exceeded expectations, and his depression resolved.

Both cases demonstrated positive outcomes, and the client satisfaction with TFT was excellent.

- *General mental illness:* A very large, although uncontrolled, study of TFT for a range of issues has suggested it may be effective.[14] This publication reviewed the SUD ratings for 714 patients who received a total of 1,594 applications of TFT. The patients had a range of psychological conditions (anxiety, adjustment disorder, pain, bereavement, depression, OCD, panic disorder, stress, phobia, PTSD), and the seven TFT therapists involved included social workers, clinical nurses, and psychologists.

  Sessions ranged between 30 and 50 minutes, and SUDs were collected as well as heart-rate variability HRV measured pre- and posttreatment regimes. The authors stated significant reductions in SUD ratings occurred within one treatment session for 31 conditions.

  This was extremely impressive and suggested the applicability of TFT across disciplines and also psychological conditions; however, the publication was not peer reviewed at the authors' request. There were no follow-up periods at all and no randomization of patients. Future studies of this size would benefit from addressing these issues to improve validity, reliability, and maintenance of effects.

Education Settings

There has been a dissertation study of TFT in an education setting that used qualitative focus group interviews.[15] The researcher was interested in what ways TFT was being used in educational settings, the effects of using it with students, and the difficulties that existed. In-depth interviews were held via telephone and e-mail with 12 adults in the United States, United Kingdom, Canada, and Mexico, who were trained in TFT and had used it with students.

Focus groups were also held with nine middle-school students between the ages of 11 and 14 who attended a community program in the northeastern part of the United States. The focus-group participants also met prior to the meeting for instruction in TFT. After using it for a week, they met in a focus group to discuss how, when, and why they used it, and their feelings about using TFT.

The student group indicated they used TFT (a) when confronted with violent situations and when they became angry, (b) when dealing with difficulties in relationships with friends and family, and (c) to help them to be better students in school. They reported that they liked TFT and found it easy to use.

The adult practitioners indicated that they used TFT with students to help them reduce stress, improve test scores, improve relationships with family and peers, reduce their feelings of violence, and improve their self-confidence. They also indicated using it for themselves, their families, and their friends to relieve stress and reduce tension. Everyone reported positive changes in students as a result of using TFT. This included improvement in behavior, self-control, attitude, and homework.

While the study focused on qualitative research only and lacked numerical data collection, and it did not investigate a comparison treatment or control group, the exploration supported the acceptance of using a tapping modality in classroom settings from both students and practitioners.

Heart Rate Variability

Dr. Roger Callahan led studies on the impact of TFT on heart rate variability (HRV). Traditionally this has been shown to be a strong predictor of mortality and is adversely affected by such problems as anxiety, depression, and trauma. Mostly these have been presented as case reports using SUD rating scales with measures of HRV.

Initially, 20 individuals with diagnosed heart problems and very low HRV received individually administered TFT.[16,17] Callahan did not describe the ECG/heart rate measurements, although he reported significant improvements in HRV (which exceeded the suggested improvements in existing literature). There wasn't a control group nor comparison treatment, and the sample size was small, but it was the start of these investigations.

Other researchers have investigated HRV with TFT as well for a wide range of issues (including phobias, anxiety, trauma, depression, fatigue, attention deficit hyperactivity disorder, learning difficulties, compulsions, obsessions, eating disorders, anger, and physical pain).[18] Thirty-nine cases from clinical practices have also indicated a lowering of SUD ratings after treatment, in most cases related to an improvement in HRV.

While these outcomes appear promising, some criticisms of these HRV studies have included strong inferences that have relied on case reports only, potentially biased samples, and lack of appropriate controls. There has also been a lack of systematic evaluation of HRV changes and flawed interpretation of HRV.[19] Therefore, further research in HRV and other physiological markers is warranted to establish the effectiveness of TFT in this area.

NOTES FROM A PRACTITIONER: TFT

Joannah Metcalfe had been successfully treating a client with a combination of aromatherapy, Reiki, and TFT; and the client was starting to feel so much better that she asked if Joannah thought her 10-year-old sister, Julie, could attend.[20] Julie was a sensitive, intelligent child, and she had begun to have an unhealthy fear of being sick—which was beginning to develop into an obsessive trait. She was very upset at the idea of being sick and had begun to restrict the variety of food she would eat, and she would not eat properly at school. She didn't want to go out to eat as a treat and was obsessing about cleanliness, especially when her mother was preparing food. If the word *sick* or *vomit* was mentioned, even on TV, she would cry and start to feel sick herself.

Julie's general practitioner had referred her to a counselor, but she was on a waiting list that was set to take at least three months, and Joannah felt concerned that this cycle was beginning to escalate. She agreed to see Julie, but suggested that her mother and sister (they are a very close family) sit in on the session too—not only to make Julie feel more at ease, but to help give information during the consultation and to benefit from the process themselves too! Joannah asked that Julie be told that her session was going to be shared by them all so that everyone could derive some benefit, as she felt Julie would feel more inclined to come and be less resistant and nervous.

Her sister confirmed that she was worried, but she did attend, and Joannah congratulated her on deciding to try something new and told her how exciting the new beginning was! Joannah then explained the whole process behind TFT, using some diagrams and a lot of very visual images. She told Julie that at some stage her brain had gotten locked into an unhelpful way of thinking about things, and all they were going to do was to help reroute the little pathways in her brain to create some new ones. This would help her remember that *sick* was just a word—like *smile* and *joy* (positive reinforcement).

Joannah also explained that brains can be viewed like a little toddler who is not happy unless they are given a little guidance and a few parameters, with lots of love. If they are given "free rein," they aren't happy and end up out of control, unhappy, and covered in mud! The aim was to allow Julie to view herself as a loving mother who is going to be gently disciplined as to where she allows her mind to go. What would she prefer to think about—a slug in a puddle or the sunshine? Joannah made Julie giggle a lot, as she felt humor to be a real key in these cases.

When Joannah was sure that they had a lovely rapport building up, and Julie was more comfortable and trusting (this took about 30 minutes and involved watching her change from sitting on the edge of her chair with hunched shoulders and shallow breaths to a more relaxed posture leaning back against the support the chair offered), they then begun using the algorithms she had chosen during the consultation. What came up were those for fear, addiction, obsession, anxiety, and panic.

After working with three of these and seeing her SUD readings drop from 9 or 10 to 1 or 0 (amidst a lot more giggling), Julie walked out looking pink of cheek and happy and relaxed.

Needless to say, when they mentioned the word *sick* before she left, she just giggled. This was *so* empowering for her, and demonstrated to her the limitless power she has to achieve what she wants when she is fully in touch with the internal resources she possesses. Her family was delighted, but Joannah thought Julie was more pleased than any of them.

Let's turn now to another technique that incorporates aspects of EFT and has emerged and been tested in research trials.

MATRIX REIMPRINTING

Matrix Reimprinting (MR) is based on the understanding that when we experience a trauma, part of our consciousness splits away into the *holographic matrix*—the energetic field that underlies all of existence. Its founder, Karl Dawson, suggests these dissociated parts become Energy Consciousness Holograms, or ECHOs.

The aim of MR is to change the habitual patterns and beliefs being held by the ECHOs in our energetic fields by working directly with the ECHOs to provide them with the resources they need to release trauma and create empowering new images to be held in our energetic fields.

MR uses EFT as part of its process and is considered a dissociative technique, which is considered favorable when working with traumatized individuals.

The First Quantitative Study of MR: Emotional Conditions

A formal EFT/MR service was set up in Sandwell, UK, in November 2010 as part of the well-being community service. A service evaluation was carried out over a 15-month period, and the researchers examined patients who had received MR.[21] This was effectively the first evaluation of MR ever published.

A total of 24 clients received MR, and 19 (79 percent) of them completed their therapy. Of these, 22 (92 percent) were female, and the average age for all clients was 47 years. The average number of sessions attended was 8.33, although the range was 3 to 49. The main presenting conditions were anxiety (14; 58.3 percent) and depression (5; 20.8 percent).

Everyone completed the CORE-10, a measure of psychological distress. It comprises a total of 10 questions covering anxiety, depression, trauma, physical problems, functioning (close relationships, social relationships), and risk to self. Higher scores indicate higher psychological distress and are categorized as "severe," "moderate severe," "moderate," "mild," or "normal." They also completed the Hospital Anxiety and Depression Scale (HADS), Rosenberg Self-Esteem Scale, and the Warwick-Edinburgh Mental Well-being Scale.

Each client was given a 10- to 15-minute introduction to EFT, then MR was incorporated during the course of therapy. Clients receiving MR were guided though the process by a therapist. Initial appointments were of up to 90 minutes' duration, with each subsequent appointment lasting up to 60 minutes.

There were statistical and significant changes for the CORE-10 (52 percent change, $p<.001$), Rosenberg Self-Esteem (46 percent change, $p<.001$), HADS Anxiety (35 percent change, $p=.007$), HADS total (34 percent change, $p=0.011$), and well-being scale (30 percent change, $p<.001$). All MR clients showed clinical improvements, and no one sought further treatment with the service.

It is worth noting, the study was small in size and did not have a control group (mainly because it was a service evaluation), and there were no long-term follow-up periods. However, just over eight clinical sessions were required, suggesting that MR may be a very cost-effective treatment.

PTSD

The first qualitative study of MR was published in 2014 and examined the impact of EFT and MR for 18 adults who were still experiencing severe emotional distress from their experiences during the 1992–95 war in Bosnia.[22] Participants had been exposed to a wide spectrum of traumatic events during the war, including beatings, confiscation or destruction of personal property, war wounds, torture, rape, sexual humiliation, and/or witnessing another person's injury or murder. There were 4 men and 10 women. Four were 30 to 40 years old, seven were 40 to 60 years old, and three were over 60 years.

Participants were assessed for PTSD symptoms using the civilian version of the PTSD Checklist (PCL-C) at baseline, immediately post-intervention and at four weeks post-intervention. Clients were also asked to fill out evaluation forms for qualitative analysis. Everyone received four individual, one-hour sessions over two weeks. Each person was also given translated written copies of the basic EFT protocol, including suggestions for using EFT to assist sleep, and were introduced to a heart-focused breathing technique.

At the start of treatment, the PTSD scores averaged 82.71; and immediately after the two weeks of MR and EFT, the average scores reduced to 53.77 (p=0.009). This was clinically and statistically significant. These scores remained stable and significant four weeks later, suggesting that the effects of MR were sustained (p=0.005).

The qualitative analysis (which was done via an evaluation form at four-week follow-up) identified the following four themes:

- Theme 1: Physical and psychological changes: "At the beginning I felt a huge burden on my shoulders, and my mind was filled with gray thoughts; but after only one session, my mind cleared, the grayness disappeared, and I felt stronger."

- Theme 2: The strength to move on and to self-care: "I managed to achieve so much within the past 10 days. Five days after the first session, I felt great and relaxed."

- Theme 3: Rapport with the MR practitioners: "I would like to express my gratefulness and thankfulness to [my therapist] . . . has made a huge positive turn in my life."

- Theme 4: Recommending it for others: "This therapy has had a positive effect on me most definitely. I would love to be able to get this kind of treatment again and I would recommend this treatment to anyone . . . I personally experienced the benefits of it."

No negative side effects were reported, and all 14 clients who completed the evaluation form gave positive feedback about their experiences. Despite the limited sample size, significant improvements were indicated; and the participants' quantitative results support the potential of MR as an effective treatment for PTSD symptoms.

NOTES FROM A PRACTITIONER: MR FOR A CHILD

The following case study was first published in the 2009 textbook *Matrix Reimprinting Using EFT* by Karl Dawson and Sasha Allenby. Here MR practitioner Carol Crowther in the UK guides Charlie through the process of working with his ECHO—the Energy Consciousness Hologram, or the part of his consciousness that froze and split off energetically into his energy field or "Matrix" at the point of a trauma.[23]

Charlie is a very likeable, sensitive, and intelligent 11-year-old. He adores playing football (soccer), is a devoted Manchester United fan, and in Carol's opinion is spiritual beyond his years.

Carol's first EFT session with Charlie was conducted during his final weeks at primary school. He had passed his 11+ (exams) and was due to start grammar school in September. He was worried about an unpleasant incident that he had had with two older local boys who would be attending his new school. They successfully used the Movie Technique in standard EFT to tap away the anxiety of the memory and also tapped on the anxiety he felt about the long bus journey he would be taking to his new school.

Charlie later attended a talk and demonstration Carol gave about EFT and displayed a poster he had drawn of the tapping points for the benefit of the members of the audience. He learned the whole process very quickly and seemed very confident in the application of EFT.

Carol's second session with Charlie was a few days before he was due to start his new school, and he was worried about his first day. Because Charlie had taken to using EFT so naturally, Carol decided to try the Matrix Reimprinting technique with him. She feels that what happened next was quite remarkable and is best expressed in Charlie's own words (and spelling) below.

Charlie's First Day Back 2 Skool

I was worried about starting my new grammar school. Carol showed me how to survive my fears, she asked me to think about a time when I felt worried. I can remember Carol asked me to think about another time when I felt frightened about going to school.

Whilst Carol tapped me, I remembered my first day at _____ Primary School. I didn't want to go. There I was sitting on the backseat behind seven-year-old Charlie, tapping him about his fears on the way in.

Carol helped me picture myself standing in the playground with my dad. I could see myself standing in my school aged 7. My dad was telling the teacher how frightened I was. I had my arms around my dad; I had my head buried in my dad's stomach. I tapped on him to get my attention, he turned around and saw me and I told him who I was. I gave him a tour of his new school whilst tapping him. I took him back into the playground and showed him to his new friends. Then I told him I was going to look after him, then he was happy. I took him back to the teacher and said good-bye. Dad had gone but he was still very happy.

Here I am now, worried about starting my secondary school and my 18-year-old self was taking me around my big new school showing me where everything was. He was looking after me for when I start. Then I'll have my 20-year-old me when I start at University!

Carol reported that the most remarkable thing about this session was that 11-year-old Charlie quite naturally took himself into the future with this technique. This was something she hadn't expected. Charlie is now settled and happy in his new school, and the transition went far more smoothly than was expected, thanks to the application of EFT and Matrix Reimprinting.

OTHER ENERGY PSYCHOLOGY TECHNIQUES

PEAT

Primordial Energy Activation and Transcendence (PEAT) is one of the newer energy psychology protocols, and in 2011 researchers examined treatment for public-speaking anxiety in 82 university students who volunteered.[24]

PEAT is based on such energy therapies as EFT, Tapas Acupressure Technique (TAT, discussed later), and other healing techniques. The creator psychologist Zivorad Slavinski says PEAT is a spiritual development system that allows a person to experience the state of non-duality. It does not lead to a cognitive understanding of non-duality, but an actual experience of the deepest set of polarities for each individual, those which they call Primes.

In this study everyone completed the Communication Anxiety Inventory Form State before and after a 20-minute PEAT treatment, and results were compared to a control group who received no treatment.

The PEAT process produced a statistically significant downward shift in communication-anxiety scores compared with the control group, with a medium effect size. An analysis of participant interviews also identified themes of effectiveness.

While further investigation is warranted, it appeared the Basic PEAT protocol was able to reduce public-speaking anxiety.

Tapas Acupressure Technique

Licensed acupuncturist Tapas Fleming developed the Tapas Acupressure Technique (TAT) in 1993 while working in the field of allergies. TAT incorporates elements of and builds on other acupressure techniques. The essence of the pose or gesture one makes while focusing on a series of statements includes cupping the occipital area on the back of the head with one hand and placing the ring finger and thumb gently into the inner canthus of each eye, while resting the ring and middle finger gently in the middle of the forehead. While many single-case studies exist supporting the TAT process for many concerns, several studies have examined it for weight-loss maintenance.

In the first, a randomized controlled trial of 92 overweight and obese adults recruited to a 12-week behavioral weight-loss program were allocated to one of three weight-loss-maintenance interventions.[25] These were qigong (QI, a breathing exercise that uses body posture and movement), TAT, and a self-directed support (SDS) group as an attention control. Eighty-eight percent of the patients completed the study.

The authors were looking for weight-loss maintenance at six months after the randomization. All patients also engaged in interviews to examine any extra benefits they received, as well as any barriers to adhering to the program. At six months, the TAT group maintained 1.2 kilograms (2.6 pounds) more weight loss than the SDS group did (p=0.09), and 2.8 kilograms (6.1 pounds) more weight loss than the QI group did (p=0.00), only regaining 0.1 kilogram (0.22 pounds).

Secondary analysis revealed that participants who had been unsuccessful at weight loss in the past were more likely to regain weight if assigned to the SDS group, but this effect was not present in the QI and TAT groups (p=0.03).

A second study involved 285 obese adults who were at least 30 years old, had a body mass index between 30 and 50 inclusive, weighed less than 181.8 kilograms (400 pounds), and lived in the Portland, Oregon, metropolitan area.[26] Of the group, 79 percent were female, and the average age was 56 years.

Everyone had completed a six-month behavioral weight-loss program prior to randomization. Those who successfully lost weight (at least 4.54 kilograms or 10 pounds) and attended more than 70 percent of the weekly group sessions were randomized into either TAT or a control intervention (social-support group meetings led by professionals).

Both groups met for 13 contact hours across eight group sessions during the six months. The main outcome was change in weight from the beginning of the weight-loss-maintenance intervention to 12 months later, but the researchers also examined changes in depression, stress, insomnia, and quality of life.

There was actually no significant difference in weight regain between the two conditions: 1.72 kilogram weight regain for TAT and 2.96 kilogram weight regain for the social-support group. However, those adults with greater initial weight loss were more likely to gain weight in the social-support group, but had less weight regain in the TAT group.

There were no differences between the two groups for the secondary outcomes of depression, stress, insomnia, and quality of life.

These studies tell us that while TAT might be promising in the area of weight-loss maintenance, more trials are needed with comparisons to gold standard approaches.

TAKE-HOME POINTS

While EFT has emerged to date with the strongest research base, other modalities also including tapping are now being published. The advantage of these approaches is that one size rarely fits all for any treatment approach. And having other options with sound research behind them then offers members of the public a sense of confidence in many methods.

I believe we will continue to see these areas evolve in the research with larger and more sophisticated clinical trials. As community awareness increases and scientific recognition grows, we may see other tapping techniques join the evidence-based field.

Chapter
11

COMMON OBSTACLES TO SUCCESS

Sometimes we hear that people have used tapping, either on their own or supported by someone, and yet very little changes. With the research and publications growing, and the positive outcomes being reported, it begs the question, *Why does it sometimes not appear to work?*

In Chapter 1 some frequently asked questions were covered, and you may want to review those again now. However, there are often other reasons tapping may not be resulting in desired outcomes. Let's have a look at potential reasons and solutions.

REASON 1: BEING TOO GLOBAL

Tapping works best when someone is very specific with their choice of words or, for example, the feeling they are focused on. Chapter 1 discussed the concept of tabletops and table legs, and that bigger, global issues often represent the top of the table. An example might be "I always run late." This would be a global issue.

Tapping just on the statement "I always run late" may not change anything in your behavior.

The table legs represent the times in your life you have run late, and some of them may have had significant consequences. Tapping on those specific times in life, memories of them or things that resulted because you ran late would have a more successful outcome.

REASON 2: THERE ARE REASONS TO KEEP THE ISSUE

At first glance this may seem strange: why would someone want to keep an issue they really wanted to change? An example might be smoking. Someone really does want to quit smoking and cannot think of any reason they want to continue. Yet tapping doesn't appear to affect anything—they keep smoking!

In this case it is often worth asking about the upside of the behavior or anything associated. This is often called secondary gain, and can even be quite unconscious (not in your awareness). If you are diligently tapping, and nothing much is changing, or your SUD rating out of 10 doesn't seem to decrease at all, you can ask these questions to see if there is any upside:

- What would it be like to have none of your symptoms/problems?

- What benefits are you getting from this illness/ behavior/problem?

- What would you have to give up if your illness/ problem went away?

- Why might you deserve this illness/problem?

REASON 3: STOPPING TOO EARLY (OR NOT EVEN STARTING)

While tapping can be a relatively quick technique compared to traditional approaches, and people might report dramatic shifts in a short period of time, this is not always the case. Tapping may need to occur regularly and over time for persistent patterns, feelings, or behavior to change. When someone reports they have done some tapping but nothing happened, it is often worth asking how long they tapped for, and what the SUD rating out of 10 was when they ceased.

Often not persisting and stopping before getting to a 0 or 1 out of 10 is a clue as to why it didn't work that time. There is no reason you can't stop tapping and come back to it another time, but the important thing to note here is that you come back, and always aim for a decrease in SUD rating to a very low number.

It would be fair to say as well that if you didn't actually ever do any tapping, it won't work. Sometimes people want to tap, but don't know where to start. So they don't start at all. If they were to just begin tapping on *any* aspect of the situation, that would start things moving.

Part of this may also be not knowing the right words to say. It is hard to get tapping wrong, but even starting with a setup statement such as "I'm afraid of getting it wrong," or "I don't know where to start" would work.

REASON 4: GOING POSITIVE TOO SOON

Because of the seemingly counterintuitive approach of stating the negative in tapping, sometimes people want to tap with positive words or affirmations. And they do this too early. Carl Jung famously said, "What you resist persists," meaning if there is a persistent feeling or belief or pattern of behavior, and this is not completely addressed—in this case, with tapping—then it is likely to continue even if you tap with positive words.

Think of it like spraying air freshener when the source of the smell is actually still in the room. Eventually you will smell it again. Positive tapping does indeed have a place, but only after the issue at hand is dealt with.

REASON 5: IGNORING THE FLEETING THOUGHTS

Sometimes when people begin tapping and are new to the process, when they have a random thought or fleeting glimpse of a memory come to mind, they ignore it.

Seasoned tappers will know that if this does happen while tapping, it may be your unconscious mind letting you know what might be underneath (or the origin of what you are tapping on). Even if the fleeting thought or passing memory appears completely unrelated, it might be worth examining.

REASON 6: IGNORING THE ASPECTS

In Chapter 1, I discussed the idea that issues can often be like a puzzle. There are many pieces, and these aspects may all need tapping on when addressing an issue. If someone taps on an issue, and it does seem to resolve, but then a week later notice something in their life or behavior that is still the same, they might think tapping didn't work. It may be that it worked on the aspect they were tapping on at the time, but a week later a slightly different aspect presented itself. This just means tapping on the new aspect. It may be faster to resolve the second time around.

An example might be that someone taps on the physical symptoms of a headache and feels fine when they finish. But a week later, they have another headache. They may be better served to tap on the underlying emotional core issues, as well as the physical symptoms. The headache may be the body's response to what is happening emotionally in their life, and that's where tapping would be better focused. It may be due to hydration or other factors as well.

REASON 7: CHANGING THE FOCUS TOO OFTEN

When an issue is quite large, it can be overwhelming when starting to tap. For example, someone may have a lifetime of emotional eating, and when they start tapping, there is a major download of thoughts, feelings, and memories. This is a lot to deal with in a single tapping session (or even many sessions!).

The risk here is that people may find themselves going down many different table legs and jumping from one thought to another, without truly getting resolution on any of them. So it seems like EFT doesn't work.

It is always a good idea to write down everything that comes to mind, but then stay focused on one area only until that SUD rating is very low (0 or 1). It will result in a better outcome. If this is difficult to do alone, working with someone who is trained and experienced is always recommended.

REASON 8: I HAVE A BELIEF (AND FEELINGS)

This reason relates somewhat to the secondary-gain reason above. Beliefs are thought patterns that have become quite permanent, and are formed early in life. We seek confirmation in our everyday life that our thoughts, and ultimately core beliefs and schemas, make sense to us (otherwise we wouldn't keep them!).

If tapping makes us question those, this can be uncomfortable (and we can become defensive). Some people enjoy being "unfixable" or being a "tough case" and unconsciously enjoy that nothing helps them. They don't want to be the same as everyone else, and they may make it difficult for anyone working with them to help. Part of addressing this involves asking whether there is an upside to being a "tough case." And what does it mean if you're not?

I have often found that people who are very skeptical of approaches such as tapping have a vested interest in *being* skeptical (rather than really rejecting tapping). For some, being skeptical is a sign of intelligence and discernment, and not being this way might mean they are gullible and naïve. These ideas can be addressed with EFT (e.g., there may be childhood memories where these decisions were made, and while they were very appropriate then, they may not serve you well now as an adult). I always wait until a client is ready to address these, as resistance may occur otherwise.

REASON 9: NOT KEEPING A RECORD

There is something unique to tapping called the Apex Effect. After all my years in traditional psychotherapy, I have never seen anything quite like this.

This phenomenon is when a client taps on an issue, achieves complete resolution, then promptly forgets it was tapping that made the difference. In my trials of food cravings, when we follow-up our participants a year later and ask them how the food craving is that they tapped on, they invariably look surprised. They tell us they never eat that food and can't recall when they last did! We remind them they tapped on that food in the clinical trial, that they were eating it several times a day. They brush this off nonchalantly and dismiss that tapping could have possibly been the reason.

So the Apex Effect refers to the notion that people do not attribute any success to EFT. They may cite other reasons such as distraction, their own willpower, time, or random other things. One way of addressing this is to keep a record of what you tap on. Keeping a journal (for example, The Tapping Journal) of the issue, setup statements, SUD ratings, and outcomes is one way to be able to look back and see what has changed.[1]

When I work with clients, I always show them the notes I wrote weeks and months earlier, when they were tapping on an issue. They are constantly surprised, and it does help with them realizing how far they have come and what has actually changed.

REASON 10: RELYING ON SCRIPTS

In our wonderful online world, and with so many people skilled in EFT offering resources and programs, there is a lot available. It is not uncommon to find example tapping scripts or setup statements available online, for a range of everyday problems. For example, if I googled how to use tapping for creating more wealth in my life, I might find scripts or videos suggesting I tap on these statements:

- Money flows to me easily (or not).

- There is plenty for everyone (or not).

- My money is an expression of my spiritual values (or not).

- Unexpected money comes to me (or not).

- I love money, and money loves me (or not).

- I live in abundance (or not).

Tapping on these topics might get me somewhere but may also not truly get to the core of why I have money concerns and don't live in abundance. The main thing to remember is that YouTube videos and scripts are an excellent starting point, but they are just that: *the starting point*. Tapping always works best when it is specific to you. That said, we do know many common issues that need to be addressed in relation to single issues or behaviors, but personalizing it all gives you the real success. Remember: tapping works best when you are very specific.

So watch and read away, but always pay attention to your own fleeting thoughts or memories that surface as you tap. Then turn your attention to those and leave the scripts alone.

COMMON MISTAKEN BELIEFS OF BEGINNERS

I want to share a fantastic list of common mistaken thoughts about EFT by expert practitioner and trainer Valerie Lis, reprinted here with her permission.[2] I couldn't write this any better.

Mistake #1: EFT works on your memories and thoughts.

EFT does not work on your memories and thoughts. It works on the *physical response* associated with your memories and thoughts.

If you have a fear of spiders, for example, there is a fight-or-flight (stress) response. Your heart rate increases, breathing accelerates, pupils dilate, and digestion stops. These symptoms occur when you think about a spider or get close to one. With tapping, there is a sudden shift from fight-or-flight to deep relaxation. As a result, your body's automated response to spiders (conditioned link) is broken, and the fear is permanently released. The memory itself remains the same. To resolve this mistake, ask before tapping: "Where do you feel this in your body?" This assures an accurate starting point to measure your progress. If you have a strong physical response, it usually means you are ready to tap. It also makes it easier to measure shifts as they occur.

Mistake #2: Emotional distress is to be avoided.

When working with EFT, emotional distress is beneficial. This is one of the hidden "secrets" in the world of tapping. When clients cry with me, I am honored and joyful. Tapping through tears produces a powerful release. It is exhilarating to connect and share this experience with my clients.

On a scale from 1 to 10, 5 to 10 is the "sweet spot." If your emotional distress is too high (i.e., higher than 10, or "out of control"), you may want to tap in silence. If you do not have emotional distress, or the level is too low, you may find it ineffective to tap. To resolve this mistake, simply focus on the emotional distress. And then tap it away.

Mistake #3: "Big" problems from long ago are more challenging to clear.

EFT is evidence-based for post-traumatic stress disorder (PTSD), phobias, and generalized anxiety (and much more). This shows that EFT is effective on intense issues. Events where there is no emotional distress are actually more challenging to clear. You should, however, protect yourself. Rather than tapping on your own to clear your big issues, you may want to work with a qualified practitioner.

Mistake #4: You must find the "right" words.

This is one of the most common mistakes among new students of EFT. Tapping scripts and tap-alongs support the belief that you must find the right words. It is actually more important to be in your "feeling space." For effective results with EFT, *it is essential to be in your feeling space.*

Mistake #5: You must always follow the "correct" procedure.

This includes stating the setup statement three times and calling out reminder phrases on the eight primary tapping points. Yes, it is important to know the correct procedures. At the same time, you should not be controlled by them. EFT is a forgiving process. In certain situations, steps can be skipped.

The purpose of the setup statement, for example, is to resolve psychological reversal. Reversals occur only 20 percent of the time and are associated with a lack of emotion.

So, especially when emotions are high, you can eliminate the setup.

In addition, individual tapping points can be skipped or missed. On occasion, reminder phrases can also be eliminated. Rather than blindly following rules for correctness, you could simply try to focus on the charge and tap the points.

Mistake #6: You must call out reminder phrases to stay focused on the memory or belief.

Rather than calling out reminder phrases to stay focused on the memory or belief, it is more important to stay in your feeling space. Overthinking, that is, being in your "head bubble," is counterproductive and slows down the process. Calling out reminder phrases may cause you to move from your feeling space back to your head bubble. If it does, reminder phrases are a distraction. Especially with high emotional intensity, you may want to avoid reminder phrases and tap in silence.

Mistake #7: You must go through the entire "story" and know how to resolve the presenting issue before you begin tapping.

It is not always necessary to understand the story or the issue. I believe that the best practice is to begin tapping as soon as possible. EFT seems to increase intuition; memories appear exactly when they are needed.

The simplest approach is to (1) find the emotional charge, (2) tap, (3) evaluate, (4) find the emotional charge, (5) tap, (6) evaluate . . . and so on. Following this process often leads to enlightened, magical, "goose bump" moments.

Mistake #8: Positives are to be avoided. Or, alternatively: Positives are to be encouraged.

The use of negatives versus positives while tapping is a common topic for discussion. I believe it is more important to determine whether the words or phrases are charged. For example, if "I am ugly" makes you emotional, this is the correct phrase. If "I am beautiful" makes you emotional, this is the correct phrase.

I have found an interesting relationship between negative self-talk and charged positives. This may provide a clue on which form should be used. Anyway, it does not matter whether words are negative or positive. If you shift your focus to charged phrases, your tapping sessions will be more productive.

Many students of EFT like to repeat blocks of affirmations while tapping. Although this does not provide deep, transitional, permanent shifts, it can be a nice tool for relaxation.

Mistake #9: Since there is a benefit to tapping on your own, there is no need to work with a practitioner.

EFT is a self-tool, so it is worthwhile to tap on your own. If you work with a qualified practitioner, though, you will likely find that your results will improve.

Mistake #10: You need to be trained in EFT. Or, alternatively: There is no need to be trained in EFT.

Proficiency falls on a continuum. On one side are those who have never been trained. As a self-help tool, it is possible to get results on your own. These results, however, often come with limitations.

Further up the spectrum are those who have been trained in the core curriculum. They get consistent results on self-work and on most issues when working with others.

The highest level includes those who get consistent results on self-work and on most issues when working with others. Their results are also faster, deeper, and more complete than other EFT practitioners.

CONCLUSION

By now it is, hopefully, glaringly obvious that EFT or tapping is a stress management or reduction tool. It is self-applied and a way of calming your body so you can think more clearly about your problem at hand.

I have heard EFT described as emotional acupuncture, emotional WD-40, and a relaxation technique. All of these are correct: we may use it in therapeutic settings, but the reality is that it is a stress-management technique. Finding a way to describe it to clients or patients, or your neighbor, may take time, and I would suggest trying a few ways to see what suits you best and how people respond. I always recommend tapping on yourself if you are worried about what people will think when you tell them about EFT. It is one of my secrets; I did this many years ago because I needed to be able to tell other researchers and staff what I was doing, and didn't want my own worries getting in the road!

I promised I would also tell you how I share this seemingly "new" technique when talking with the media and other professionals. I have always found that building a bridge to what they might already accept is paramount.

If I am speaking with other professionals, I might say: EFT or tapping is a brief, novel intervention combining elements of exposure and cognitive therapy and somatic stimulation. It is often referred to as "psychological acupuncture" and uses a two-finger tapping process with a cognitive statement.

This sounds like a mouthful, but it speaks to people who use cognitive therapies, and doesn't seem too far removed from what they already know. I share that it is *very* similar to exposure therapy used in anxiety disorders, OCD, phobias . . . except the "response prevention" aspect is the tapping in EFT (rather than deep breathing or muscle contractions). I also highlight somatic elements that are used in other therapies (e.g., dialectical behavior therapy for borderline personality disorder patients and weighted items like blankets for autism sufferers). In essence I am building a bridge to what they already know and accept.

Any of the above can be used when talking to the media, but they often respond well to the concept that EFT is a psychological form of acupuncture. We just use a tapping process on acupoints instead of a needle. They also enjoy statistics such as this: EFT belongs to a group called "energy psychology," and it has over 100 research studies, review articles, and meta-analyses published in professional, peer-reviewed journals.

Above all, enjoy sharing the news of this exciting research. The numbers keep growing, and the evidence is actually there. Sometimes the real question is: how *much* evidence do you need?

When I received the invitation to write this book, I had more than one moment of quiet panic. To bring together the field of EFT research in an easy-to-read manner, and to do justice to describing what researchers have completed, was difficult at times. I know how challenging research trials are to conduct, and follow-up periods are even harder, and I truly hope I have represented everyone's efforts in a respectful and honest light. I love being a researcher and conducting trials myself, and I have been in awe writing this book at how much is being achieved in this field. I thought I knew of most of the published research, but I discovered treasures along the way!

My suggestions from this point forward would be to stay abreast of the research as it is released and stay open to the possibilities that fourth-wave approaches such as EFT may become standard practice in years to come. The distinct advantages EFT enjoys over other methodologies not only include features such as brevity and long-term sustainability but also the client stories that present a picture of true healing and emotional freedom. Research outcomes are only one half of the coin—the other side is the lived experience. When positive patient outcomes are parallel to the statistical significance levels, then we know we indeed have a complete process.

It has been my absolute pleasure to guide you through this journey, and I look forward to hearing your own stories and outcomes.

Stay open.

RESOURCES

．．．

For information about EFT, including a free downloadable Get Started package, go to www.eftuniverse.com. You'll find thousands of case histories of people who've used EFT successfully for every conceivable problem. You'll also find practitioner listings, tutorials, books, DVDs, classes, volunteer opportunities, and other resources to allow you to get the most from EFT.

You could consider taking a live hands-on Clinical EFT workshop to experience the technique yourself. Always know you can also consult a Clinical EFT practitioner. Many of them offer free initial consultations so you can determine if they're a fit for you. You might find talking to a skilled practitioner helps resolve things quicker and more easily than tapping on your own.

WHERE TO FIND MORE RESEARCH ON EFT

While this book has presented the best of the best research out there and highlighted emerging areas, there is a plethora of case reports and pilot studies not covered here. Here are some of the most comprehensive websites to explore and follow for future research:

- **Dr. Craig Weiner and Alina Frank**, EFT trainers and producers of *The Science of Tapping* documentary maintain a very comprehensive overview of EFT and tapping research here: www.efttappingtraining.com/eft-research.

- **EFT Universe**, one of the most-visited alternative-health websites, maintains research here: www.eftuniverse.com/research-studies/eft-research.

- **EFT International (previously known as The Association for the Advancement of Meridian Energy Techniques)** is a voluntary, not-for-profit association committed to advancing and upholding the highest standards for education; training; professional development; and promotion of the skillful, creative, and ethical application of EFT. They maintain their research here: https://aametinternational.org/discover-eft/eft-science-research.

- **The Association for Comprehensive Energy Psychology (ACEP)** is a professional organization for licensed health-care providers and allied health disciplines that serves to organize and unify energy psychology methods, provides professional support and education, and establishes ethical guidance in practice. They present a range of research, including other energy psychology research, here: www.energypsych.org/?Research_Landing.

- **My own research** is maintained through Bond University's research portal, and my professional research page is here: https://research.bond.edu.au/en/persons/peta-stapleton.

THE BEST RESEARCHERS IN THE FIELD

Here is a list, although not exhaustive, of EFT giants to follow:

- **Dr. Peta Stapleton** is Australia's leading EFT researcher and academic. Peta is also a trainer and leads teams bringing EFT into schools, corporate settings, and

the community. www.petastapleton.com and www.
evidencebasedeft.com

- **Alina Frank** has conducted EFT trainings throughout
  the United States, Canada, and Mexico and has
  received five-star ratings for those trainings from
  Tapping International, Yelp, Google Plus Places, and
  EFT Universe. She has also conducted EFT Matrix
  Reimprinting trainings throughout the United States,
  Canada, Israel, and Mexico. Alina is the founder
  and current organizer of the annual NW Tappers
  Gathering, offers free EFT to emergency responders
  through Whidbey CareNet, and was a master presenter
  for the Warriors Wellness Project's Trauma Tune-Up.
  www.efttappingtraining.com

- **Dr. Craig Weiner** is a chiropractor and international
  trainer in EFT and Matrix Reimprinting and trauma
  work and trains with his wife, Alina (above). He is
  the producer and director of the Matrix Reimprinting
  EFT World Summit, and with Alina has produced
  the documentary film *The Science of Tapping*. www.
  efttappingtraining.com

- **Carol Look** is an intuitive energy healer,
  psychotherapist, and EFT Master. www.carollook.com

- **Margaret Lynch** is a transformational speaker, coach,
  and author. www.margaretmlynch.com

- **Jack Canfield** is co-author of the number-one *New
  York Times* best-selling *Chicken Soup for the Soul* series,
  which has sold more than 500 million copies in 47
  languages. He has co-written a book on EFT for success
  with Pamela Bruner. www.tappingintoultimatesuccess.
  com and www.JackCanfield.com

- **Pamela Bruner** is a success coach and co-wrote a
  success and EFT book with Jack Canfield. www.
  makeyoursuccessreal.com

- **Dr. Dawson Church** is an award-winning author (www.genieinyourgenes.com) and maintains EFTuniverse.com. www.dawsonchurch.com

- **Nick Ortner** is a *New York Times* best-selling Hay House author of several EFT books and producer of *The Tapping Solution* documentary. www.thetappingsolution.com

- **Jessica Ortner** is the author of the Hay House book *The Tapping Solution for Weight Loss & Body Confidence* and producer of *The Tapping Solution*. She is also the host of The Tapping World Summit, an annual online event that has attracted more than 500,000 attendees from around the world. www.jessicaortner.com

- **Karl Dawson** is one of only 28 EFT Masters worldwide and an international EFT trainer and presenter. www.matrixreimprinting.com

- **Dr. Patricia Carrington** is a leading psychologist and pioneer in energy psychology and modern meditation. She is a widely acclaimed author, researcher, and innovator in energy-related self-development methods, and one of a few EFT practitioners worldwide to have earned the designation of Founding EFT Master from EFT's originator, Gary Craig. www.patcarrington.com

- **Dr. David Feinstein** is a clinical psychologist and internationally recognized leader in the rapidly emerging field of energy psychology. His scientific papers have provided a foundation for understanding how it is possible to quickly and noninvasively alter brain chemistry for therapeutic gain. His popular, award-winning books have opened the approach to many. www.innersource.net/ep

- **Dr. Lori Leyden** is a trauma-healing professional known internationally for using EFT/tapping in her work with hundreds of orphan genocide survivors in

Rwanda. She was the leader of The Tapping Solution Foundation's humanitarian work that supported those affected by the Sandy Hook Elementary School tragedy. www.createglobalhealing.org

- **Gene Monterastelli** hosts Tapping Q & A. On this site, you will find over 500 free tapping- and EFT-related resources, including a regular podcast. www.tappingqanda.com

OTHER EFT TOOLS

- **toolboxtime** is best described as your "go to" with simple suggestions to assist you with day-to-day emotional and physical challenges. Focusing on four key energy therapies—EFT, essential oils, light therapy, and intentions—to use in your own home, this easy-to-understand and easy-to-navigate reference deck has been developed in collaboration with experts in the field. It contains 42 cards covering five key emotions, 30 common symptoms, seven information cards, and an information booklet in a durable box with tabbed dividers. www.toolboxtime.com

- **EFT Radio Online** is a dedicated space for interviews with pioneers and leaders. www.eftradioonline.com

ENDNOTES

....

Introduction

1. Shapiro, Francine. *Eye Movement Desensitization and Reprocessing (EMDR): Basic Principles, Protocols, and Procedures.* 2nd ed. New York: The Guilford Press, 2001.

2. "How Common Is PTSD?" *PTSD: National Center for PTSD.* U.S. Department of Veteran Affairs. October 3, 2016. https://www.ptsd.va.gov/public/ptsd-overview/basics/how-common-is-ptsd.asp.

3. "About ADAA: Facts & Statistics." Anxiety and Depression Association of America. https://www.adaa.org/about-adaa/press-room/facts-statistics.

4. "Investing in Treatment for Depression and Anxiety Leads to Fourfold Return." World Health Organization. April 13, 2016. http://www.who.int/mediacentre/news/releases/2016/depression-anxiety-treatment/en.

5. "'Depression: Let's Talk' Says WHO, as Depression Tops List of Causes of Ill Health." World Health Organization. March 30, 2017. http://www.who.int/news-room/detail/30-03-2017-depression-let-s-talk-says-who-as-depression-tops-list-of-causes-of-ill-health.

Chapter 1

1. Energy Healing with Dr. Patricia Carrington. https://patcarrington.com.

2. Feinstein, David. "Acupoint stimulation in treating psychological disorders: Evidence of efficacy." *Review of General Psychology* 16 (2012): 364–380.

3. Dhond, R., Kettner, N., and Napadow, V. "Neuroimaging acupuncture effects in the human brain." *The Journal of Alternative and Complementary Medicine* 1, no. 6 (2007): 603–616.

4. Feinstein, David. "Rapid treatment of PTSD: Why psychological exposure with acupoint tapping may be effective." *Psychotherapy: Theory, Research, Practice, Training* 47, no. 3 (2010): 385–402.

5. Rowe, Jack. "The effects of EFT on long-term psychological symptoms." *Counseling and Clinical Psychology Journal* 2, no. 3 (2005): 104.

6. Craig, Gary et al. "Emotional Freedom Techniques (EFT) For Traumatic Brain Injury." *International Journal of Healing and Caring* 9, no. 2 (May 2009): 1–12.

Chapter 2

1. Keown, Daniel. *The Spark in the Machine: How the Science of Acupuncture Explains the Mysteries of Western Medicine.* London: Singing Dragon, 2014.

2. Lin Y-C. "Perioperative usage of acupuncture." *Pediatric Anesthesia* 16, no. 3 (2006): 231–235.

3. Santa Ana, C.F. "The adoption of complementary and alternative medicine by hospitals: A framework for decision making." *Journal Healthcare Management,* 46 (2001): 250–60.

4. McDonald, John, and Stephen Janz. *The Acupuncture Evidence Project: A Comparative Literature Review (Revised Edition).* Brisbane: Australian Acupuncture and Chinese Medicine Association Ltd, 2017. http://www.acupuncture.org.au.

5. Australian Government National Health and Medical Research Council. *NHMRC additional levels of evidence and grades for recommendations for developers of guidelines.* Australia: National Health and Medical Research Council, 2009.

6. Balshem, H. et al. "GRADE guidelines: 3. Rating the quality of evidence." *Journal of Clinical Epidemiology* 64, no. 4 (2011): 401–6.

7. McDonald, John, and Stephen Janz. *The Acupuncture Evidence Project: A Comparative Literature Review (Revised Edition)*. Brisbane: Australian Acupuncture and Chinese Medicine Association Ltd, 2017. http://www.acupuncture.org.au.

8. Craig, Gary. *The EFT Manual*. 2nd ed. Santa Rosa, CA: Energy Psychology Press, 2011.

9. Church, Dawson. *The EFT Manual*. 3rd ed. Fulton, CA: Energy Psychology Press, 2013.

10. Church, Dawson et al. "Empirically supported psychological treatments: The challenge of evaluating clinical innovations." *Journal of Nervous and Mental Disease* 202, no. 10 (2014): 699–709.

Chapter 3

1. Wampold, Bruce. *The Great Psychotherapy Debate: Model, Methods, and Findings*. Mahwah, NJ: Lawrence Erlbaum Associates, 2001.

2. Arkowitz, Hal, and Scott O. Lilienfeld. "Psychotherapy on Trial." *Scientific American Mind* 17, no. 2 (April/May 2006): 42–49.

3. Wampold, Bruce. "How important are the common factors in psychotherapy? An update." *World Psychiatry* 14, no. 3 (2015): 270–277. doi:10.1002/wps.20238.

4. Feinstein, David. "Energy Psychology: Efficacy, speed, mechanisms." *Explore: The Journal of Science and Healing* (2018): doi:10.1016/j.explore.2018.11.003.

5. Feinstein, David. "How energy psychology changes deep emotional learnings." *The Neuropsychotherapist* 10 (January 2015): 1–11.

6. Van der Kolk, Bessel. "Posttraumatic stress disorder and the nature of trauma." *Dialogues in Clinical Neuroscience* 2, no.1 (2000): 7–22.

7. Church, Dawson, Yount, Garret, and Brooks, Audrey. "The effect of emotional freedom techniques on stress biochemistry: A randomized controlled trial." *Journal of Nervous and Mental Disease* 200 (2012): 89–896.

8. Lambrou, P. T., Pratt, G. J., and Chevalier, G. "Physiological and psychological effects of a mind/body therapy on

claustrophobia." *Subtle Energies & Energy Medicine* 14, no. 3 (2003): 239–251.

9. Swingle, P. G., Pulos, L., and Swingle, M. K. "Neurophysio-logical indicators of EFT treatment of post-traumatic stress." *Subtle Energies & Energy Medicine* 15, no. 1 (2004): 75–86.

10. Fang, J. et al. "The salient characteristics of the central effects of acupuncture needling: Limbic-paralimbic-neocortical net-work modulation." *Human Brain Mapping* 30 (2009): 1196–1206. doi:10.1002/hbm.20583.

11. Napadow, V. et al. "Hypothalamus and amygdala response to acupuncture stimuli in carpal tunnel syndrome." *Pain* 130 (2007): 254–266.

12. Stapleton, Peta et al. "Neural Changes in Overweight Adults with Food Cravings after Emotional Freedom Techniques Treatment: A Feasibility Study." *OBM Integrative and Comple-mentary Medicine* (2018), under review.

13. Maharaj, M. E. "Differential gene expression after Emotional Freedom Techniques (EFT) treatment: A novel pilot protocol for salivary mRNA assessment." *Energy Psychology: Theory, Research, and Treatment* 8, no.1 (2016): 17–32. doi:10.9769/EPJ.2016.8.1.MM.

14. Church, Dawson et al. "Epigenetic effects of PTSD remedi-ation in veterans using Clinical Emotional Freedom Tech-niques: A randomized controlled pilot study." *American Journal of Health Promotion* 32, no. 1 (2018): 112–122. doi:10.1177/0890117116661154.

15. Bach, Donna et al. "Clinical EFT (Emotional Freedom Tech-niques) Improves Multiple Physiological Markers of Health." (2018), *Journal of Evidence-Based Integrative Medicine,* in press.

16. Kazantzis, N., Deane, F. P., and Ronan, K. R. "Home-work assignments in cognitive and behavioral therapy: A meta-analysis." *Clinical Psychology: Science & Practice* 7, no. 2 (2000):189–202. doi:10.1093/clipsy/7.2.189.

17. Mausbach, Brent T. et al. "The relationship between home-work compliance and therapy outcomes: An updated meta-analysis." *Cognitive Therapy and Research* 34, no. 5 (2010): 429–438.

18. Helbig, S. and Fehm, L. "Problems with homework in CBT: Rare exception or rather frequent?" *Behavioral and Cognitive Psychotherapy* 32, no. 3 (2004): 291–301. doi:10.1017/S1352465804001365.

19. Kazantzis, N., Lampropoulos, G.K., and Deane, F. P. "A national survey of practicing psychologists' use and attitudes toward homework in psychotherapy." *Journal of Consulting and Clinical Psychology* 73, no. 4 (August 2005): 742–748.

20. Feinstein, David. "Acupoint stimulation in treating psychological disorders: Evidence of efficacy." *Review of General Psychology* 16, no. 4 (2012): 364–380. doi:10.1037/a0028602.

21. Church, Dawson. "Clinical EFT (Emotional Freedom Techniques) as single session therapy: Cases, research, indications, and cautions." In M. Hoyt and M. Talmon, eds., *Capturing the Moment: Single Session Therapy and Walk-in Service*. Bethel, CT: Crown House, 2013.

22. Church, D., Geronilla, L., and Dinter, I. "Psychological symptom change in veterans after six sessions of EFT (Emotional Freedom Techniques): An observational study." *International Journal of Healing and Caring* 9, no. 1 (2009): 1–13.

23. Geronilla, L. et al. "EFT (Emotional Freedom Techniques) remediates PTSD and psychological symptoms in veterans: A randomized controlled replication trial." *Energy Psychology: Theory, Research, and Treatment* 8, no. 2 (2016): 29–41.

24. Andrade, J., and Feinstein, D. "Energy psychology: Theory, indications, evidence." In David Feinstein, *Energy Psychology Interactive* (Appendix, 199–214). Ashland, OR: Innersource, 2004.

25. Benor, Dan et al. "Pilot study of Emotional Freedom Technique (EFT), Wholistic Hybrid derived from EMDR and EFT (WHEE) and Cognitive Behavioral Therapy (CBT) for treatment of test anxiety in university students." *Explore: The Journal of Science and Healing* 5, no. 6 (2009): 338–340.

26. Hui, K. K. S. et al. "Acupuncture modulates the limbic system and subcortical gray structures of the human brain: Evidence from fMRI studies in normal subjects." *Human Brain Mapping* 9 (2000): 13–25. doi:10.1002/(SICI)1097-0193(2000)9:1<13::AID-HBM2>3.0.CO;2-F.

27. Feinstein, David. "How energy psychology changes deep emotional learnings." *The Neuropsychotherapist* 10 (January 2015), 1–11.

28. Ecker, B., Ticic, R., and Hulley, L. *Unlocking the Emotional Brain: Eliminating Symptoms at Their Roots Using Memory Reconsolidation.* New York: Routledge, 2012.

29. Nader, Karim. "Memory traces unbound." *Trends in Neurosciences* 26, no. 2 (2003): 65–72.

30. Church, Dawson. *The EFT Manual.* 3rd ed. Fulton, CA: Energy Psychology Press, 2013.

31. Feinstein, David. "Acupoint stimulation in treating psychological disorders: Evidence of efficacy." *Review of General Psychology* 16 (2012): 364–380. doi:10.1037/a0028602.

32. APA Presidential Task Force on Evidence-Based Practice. "Evidence-based practice in psychology." *American Psychologist* 61 (2006): 271-285. https://www.div12.org/psychological-treatments.

33. Church, Dawson et al. "Empirically supported psychological treatments: The challenge of evaluating clinical innovations." *Journal of Nervous and Mental Disease* 202, no. 10 (2014): 699–709.

34. Institute of Medicine. *Crossing the quality chasm: A new health system for the 21st century/Committee on Quality Health Care in America.* Washington, D.C.: The National Academies Press, 2001. https://www.nap.edu/read/10027/chapter/1#ii.

35. Waite, L. W. and Holder M. D. "Assessment of the emotional freedom technique: An alternative treatment for fear." *The Scientific Review of Mental Health Practice* 2, no. 1 (2003): 20–26.

36. Fox, L. "Is acupoint tapping an active ingredient or an inert placebo in Emotional Freedom Techniques (EFT)? A randomized controlled dismantling study." *Energy Psychology: Theory, Research, and Treatment* 5, no. 2 (2013): 15–28.

37. Rogers, R., and Sears, S. R. "Emotional Freedom Techniques for stress in students: A randomized controlled dismantling study." *Energy Psychology: Theory, Research, and Treatment* 7, no. 2 (2015): 26–32.

38. Reynolds, A. E. "Is acupoint stimulation an active ingredient in Emotional Freedom Techniques (EFT)? A controlled trial of teacher burnout." *Energy Psychology: Theory, Research, and Treatment* 7, no. 1 (2015): 14–21. doi:10.9769/EPJ.2015.07.01.AR.

39. Church, D., Stapleton, P., Yang, A., and Gallo, F. "Is tapping on acupuncture points an active ingredient in emotional freedom techniques? A systematic review and meta-analysis of comparative studies." *The Journal of Nervous and Mental Disease* 206, no. 10 (2018): 783–93. doi:10.1097/ NMD.0000000000000878.

40. Stapleton, Peta et al. "Secondary psychological outcomes in a controlled trial of emotional freedom techniques and cognitive behaviour therapy in the treatment of food cravings." *Complementary Therapies in Clinical Practice* 28 (2016): 136–145. doi:10.1016/j.ctcp.2017.06.004.

41. Cohen, Jacob. *Statistical Power Analysis for the Behavioral Sciences.* 2nd ed. Mahwah, NJ: Lawrence Erlbaum Associates (Routledge), 1988.

Chapter 4

1. National Center for PTSD. "Basic Symptoms of PTSD." *U.S. Department of Veterans Affairs.* August 13, 2015. https://www. ptsd.va.gov/public/ptsd-overview/basics/symptoms_of_ptsd. asp.

2. American Psychiatric Association. *Diagnostic and Statistical Manual of Mental Disorders.* 5th ed. Washington, DC: American Psychiatric Publishing, 2013.

3. American Psychiatric Association. "What is posttraumatic stress disorder?" January 2017. https://www.psychiatry.org/ patients-families/ptsd/what-is-ptsd.

4. Nebraska Department of Veterans' Affairs. "What is PTSD?" November 13, 2017. http://www.ptsd.ne.gov/what-is-ptsd. html.

5. Church, Dawson. "The treatment of combat trauma in veterans using EFT (Emotional Freedom Techniques): A Pilot Protocol." *Traumatology* 16, no.1 (March 2010): 55–65.

6. Church, D., Geronilla, L., and Dinter, I. "Psychological symptom change in veterans after six sessions of EFT (Emotional Freedom Techniques): An observational study." *International Journal of Healing and Caring* 9, no. 1 (2009): 1–13.

7. Church, Dawson et al. "Psychological trauma symptom improvement in veterans using emotional freedom techniques: A randomized controlled trial." *Journal of Nervous & Mental Disease* 201 (2013): 153–160.

8. Geronilla, L. et al. "EFT (Emotional Freedom Techniques) remediates PTSD and psychological symptoms in veterans: A randomized controlled replication trial." *Energy Psychology: Theory, Research, and Treatment* 8, no. 2 (2016): 29–41.

9. Church, Dawson and Brooks, Audrey. "CAM and energy psychology techniques remediate PTSD symptoms in veterans and spouses." *Explore: The Journal of Science and Healing* 10 (2014): 24–33.

10. Church, D., Sparks, T., and Clond, M. "EFT (Emotional Freedom Techniques) and resiliency in veterans at risk for PTSD: A randomized controlled trial." *Explore: The Journal of Science and Healing* 12, no. 5 (2016): 355–365.

11. Stein, P. and Brooks, A. "Efficacy of EFT provided by coaches versus licensed therapists in veterans with PTSD." *Energy Psychology Journal: Theory, Research & Treatment* 3 (2011). doi:10.9769/EPJ.2011.3.1.PKS.

12. Hartung, J., and Stein, P. "Telephone delivery of EFT (emotional freedom techniques) remediates PTSD symptoms in veterans." *Energy Psychology Journal: Theory, Research & Treatment* 4 (2011): 33-40.

13. Karatzias, T. et al. "A controlled comparison of the effectiveness and efficiency of two psychological therapies for post-traumatic stress disorder: Eye movement desensitization and reprocessing vs. emotional freedom techniques." *Journal of Nervous & Mental Disease* 199, no. 6 (2011): 372–378.

14. Al-Hadethe, A., Hunt, N., Al-Qaysi, G., and Thomas, S. "Randomised controlled study comparing two psychological therapies for post-traumatic stress disorder (PTSD): Emotional freedom techniques (EFT) vs. narrative exposure therapy

(NET)." *Journal of Traumatic Stress Disorders and Treatment* 4, no. 4 (2015): 1–12. doi:10.4172/2324-8947.1000145.

15. Nemiro, A. and Papworth, S. "Efficacy of two evidence-based therapies, Emotional Freedom Techniques (EFT) and Cognitive Behavioral Therapy (CBT) for the treatment of gender violence in the Congo: A randomized controlled trial." *Energy Psychology: Theory, Research, and Treatment* 7, no. 2 (2015): 13–25. doi:10.9769/EPJ.2015.7.2.AN.

16. Metcalf, O. et al. "Efficacy of fifteen emerging interventions for the treatment of post-traumatic stress disorder: A systematic review." *Journal of Traumatic Stress* 29, no. 1 (2016): 88–92. doi:10.1002/jts.22070.

17. Sebastian, B., and Nelms, J. "The effectiveness of emotional freedom techniques in the treatment of post-traumatic stress disorder: A meta-analysis." *Explore: The Journal of Science and Healing* 13 (2017): 16–25. doi:10.1016/j.explore.2016.10.001.

18. Church, Dawson and David Feinstein. "The manual stimulation of acupuncture points in the treatment of post-traumatic stress disorder: A review of clinical emotional freedom techniques." *Medical Acupuncture* 29, no. 4 (2017): 249–253.

19. Swingle, P., Pulos, L., and Swingle, M. K. "Neurophysiological indicators of EFT treatment of post-traumatic stress." *Journal of Subtle Energies & Energy Medicine* 15 (2005): 75–86.

20. Gurret, J. M. et al. "Post-earthquake rehabilitation of clinical PTSD in Haitian seminarians." *Energy Psychology: Theory, Research, and Treatment* 4, no. 2 (2012): 26–34.

21. Lubin, H. and Schneider, T. "Change is possible: EFT (Emotional Freedom Techniques) with life-sentence and veteran prisoners at San Quentin State Prison." *Energy Psychology: Theory, Research, & Treatment* 1, no.1 (2009): 83–88.

22. Church, Dawson et al. "Single session reduction of the intensity of traumatic memories in abused adolescents after EFT: A randomized controlled pilot study." *Traumatology* 18 (2012): 73–79. http://dx.doi.org/10.1177/1534765611426788.

23. Feinstein, David. "Rapid treatment of PTSD: Why psychological exposure with acupoint tapping may be effective." *Psychotherapy: Theory, Research, Practice, and Training* 47, no. 3 (2010): 385–402.

24. Kalla, Mahima and Peta Stapleton. "How emotional freedom techniques (EFT) may be utilizing memory reconsolidation mechanisms for therapeutic change in neuropsychiatric disorders such as PTSD and phobia: A proposed model." *European Journal of Neuroscience* (under review 2019).

25. Ecker, B., Ticic, R., and Hulley, L. *Unlocking the Emotional Brain: Eliminating Symptoms at Their Roots Using Memory Reconsolidation.* New York: Routledge, 2012.

26. Nader, Karim. "Memory traces unbound." *Trends in Neurosciences* 26, no. 2 (2003): 65–72.

27. Church, Dawson. "Emotional freedom techniques to treat post-traumatic stress disorder in veterans: Review of the evidence, survey of practitioners, and proposed clinical guidelines." *The Permanente Journal* 21 (2017): 16–100. doi:10.7812/TPP/16-100.

28. Weathers, F. W. et al. "PTSD Checklist for DSM-5 (PCL-5)." National Center for PTSD. U.S. Department of Veterans Affairs. May 11, 2017.

29. Craig, Gary. "BATTLE TAP Protocol." Accessed October 13, 2017. http://battletap.org/Protocol.aspx.

30. Rosenthal, Michele. "If you have PTSD you should know immediately: You are not alone." Heal My PTSD with Michele Rosenthal. Accessed August 28, 2017, http://www.healmyptsd.com/education/post-traumatic-stress-disorder-statistics.

31. Church, Dawson. "Veterans Administration Approves EFT (Emotional Freedom Techniques) Treatment." *The Huffington Post.* October 17, 2017. https://www.huffingtonpost.com/entry/veterans-administration-approves-eft-emotional-freedom_us_597fc82ee4b0cb4fc1c73be2.

Chapter 5

1. Lazarus, R. S. and Folkman, S. *Stress, Appraisal, and Coping.* New York: Springer, 1984.

2. Church, Dawson, Yount, Garret, and Brooks, Audrey. "The effect of emotional freedom techniques (EFT) on stress

biochemistry: A randomized controlled trial." *Journal of Nervous and Mental Disease* 200 (2012): 891–896.

3. Rowe, Jack. "The effects of EFT on long-term psychological symptoms." *Counseling and Clinical Psychology Journal* 2 (2005): 104.

4. Church, Dawson and Brooks, Audrey. "The effect of a brief EFT (Emotional Freedom Techniques) self-intervention on anxiety, depression, pain and cravings in health-care workers." *Integrative Medicine: A Clinician's Journal* 9, no. 4 (2010): 40–44.

5. Stewart, Anthony et al. "Can Emotional Freedom Techniques (EFT) be effective in the treatment of emotional conditions? Results of a service evaluation in Sandwell." *Journal of Psychological Therapies in Primary Care* 2 (2013): 71–84.

6. The Anxiety and Depression Association of America. Accessed October 15, 2017. https://adaa.org.

7. Andrade, Joaquin and Feinstein, David. "Energy psychology: Theory, indications, evidence." In David Feinstein, *Energy Psychology Interactive* (Appendix 199–214). Ashland, OR: Innersource, 2004.

8. Andrade, Joaquin and Feinstein, David. "Preliminary report of the first large scale study of energy psychology." In David Feinstein, *Energy Psychology Interactive*. Ashland, OR: Innersource, 2004.

9. "The Neurological Foundations of Energy Psychology: Brain Scan Changes During 4 Weeks of Treatment for Generalized Anxiety Disorder." *Energy Psychology: Easily Learn EFT & Related Methods*. http://www.innersource.net/ep/articlespublished/neurological-foundations.html.

10. Bougea, A. M et al. "Effect of the emotional freedom technique on perceived stress, quality of life, and cortisol salivary levels in tension-type headache sufferers: A randomized controlled trial." *Explore: The Journal of Science and Healing* 9, no. 2 (2013): 91–99. doi:10.1016/j.explore.2012.12.005.

11. Temple, G., and Mollon, P. "Reducing Anxiety in Dental Patients using EFT: A Pilot Study." *Energy Psychology: Theory, Research and Treatment* 3, no. 2 (2011): 53–56.

12. Cartland, Angela. "Emotional freedom techniques (EFT) remediates dental fear: A case series." *Energy Psychology: Theory, Research, and Treatment* 8, no. 2 (2016): 42–66.

13. Saleh, B., Tiscione, M., and Freedom, John. "The effect of emotional freedom techniques on patients with dental anxiety: A pilot study." *Energy Psychology: Theory, Research, and Treatment* 9, no. 1 (2017): 26–38. doi:10.9769/EPJ.2017.9.1.BS.

14. Patterson, S. L. "The effect of emotional freedom technique on stress and anxiety in nursing students: A pilot study." *Nurse Education Today* 40 (2016): 104–110.

15. Thomas, R. M., Cutinho, S. P., and Aranha, D. M. S. "Emotional Freedom Techniques (EFT) reduces anxiety among women undergoing surgery." *Energy Psychology: Theory, Research, and Treatment* 9, no.1 (2017): 18–25. doi:10.9769/EPJ.2017.9.1.RT.

16. Jones, S. J., Thornton, J. A., and Andrews, H. B. "Efficacy of emotional freedom techniques (EFT) in reducing public speaking anxiety: A randomized controlled trial." *Energy Psychology: Theory, Research, and Treatment* 3, no. 1 (2011): 19–32. doi:10.9769/EPJ.2011.3.1.SJJ.JAT.HBA.

17. Christina, D. et al. "Stress management for the treatment of sleep disorders in lawyers: Pilot experimental study in Athens, Hellas." *Journal of Sleep Disorders: Treatment and Care* 5, no. 2 (2016). doi:10.4172/2325-9639.1000171.

18. Clond, M. "Emotional freedom techniques for anxiety: A systematic review with meta-analysis." *Journal of Nervous and Mental Disease* 204 (2016): 388–395. doi:10.1097/NMD.0000000000000483.

19. Freedom, John. Adapted from "EFT clears an obsessive dental phobia." *The Gary Craig Official EFT Training Centers*. Accessed January 2, 2018. https://www.emofree.com/fears-phobias/illness-death/dental-phobia-relief-john-article.html.

20. McGonigal, Kelly. *The Upside of Stress*. New York: Avery Publishing Group, 2015.

Chapter 6

1. Kessler R. C. et al. "The epidemiology of major depressive disorder: Results from the National Comorbidity Survey Replication (NCS-R)." *JAMA* 289, no. 23 (2003): 3095–3105.

2. Church, Dawson, De Asis, Midanelle, and Brooks, Audrey. "Brief group intervention using emotional freedom techniques for depression in college students: A randomized controlled trial." *Depression Research and Treatment* (2012) .doi:10.1155/2012/257172.

3. Stapleton, Peta et al. "A feasibility study: Emotional freedom techniques for depression in Australian adults." *Current Research in Psychology* 5 (2014): 19–33.

4. Chatwin, Hannah et al. "The effectiveness of cognitive behavioral therapy and emotional freedom techniques in reducing depression and anxiety among adults: A pilot study." *Integrative Medicine* 15, no. 2 (2016): 27–34.

5. Bjorntorp, P. "Do stress reactions cause abdominal obesity and comorbidities?" *Obesity Reviews* 2, no. 2 (2001): 73–86.

6. Holsboer, F. "The corticosteroid receptor hypothesis of depression," *Neuropsychopharmacology* 23, no. 5 (2000): 477–501.

7. Stapleton, Peta et al. (2013). "Depression symptoms improve after successful weight loss with emotional freedom techniques." *ISRN Psychiatry* 2013: 573532. doi:10.1155/2013/573532.

8. Nelms, J. and Castel, D. "A systematic review and meta-analysis of randomized and non-randomized trials of emotional freedom techniques (EFT) for the treatment of depression." *Explore: The Journal of Science and Healing* 12 (2016): 416–426. doi:10.1016/j.explore.2016.08.001.

Chapter 7

1. Australian Bureau of Statistics. "National Health Survey: First Results, 2014–15." December 8, 2015. http://www.abs.gov.au/ausstats/abs@.nsf/mf/4364.0.55.001.

2. Australia's Adult Health Tracker. "A report card on preventable chronic diseases, conditions and their risk factors Tracking progress for a healthier Australia by 2025." 2016. https://trove.nla.gov.au/version/235292564.

3. "Obesity and Overweight." World Health Organization. February 16, 2018. http://www.who.int/news-room/fact-sheets/detail/obesity-and-overweight.

4. Stapleton, Peta et al. "A randomized clinical trial of a meridian-based intervention for food cravings with six-month follow-up." *Behaviour Change* 28 (2011): 1–16. doi:10.1375/bech.28.1.1.

5. Stapleton, Peta et al. "Food for thought: A randomized controlled trial of emotional freedom techniques and cognitive behavioral therapy in the treatment of food cravings." *Applied Psychology: Health and Well-Being* 8 (2016): 232–257. doi:10.1111/aphw.12070.

6. Stapleton., Peta et al. "Secondary psychological outcomes in a controlled trial of Emotional Freedom Techniques and cognitive behavior therapy in the treatment of food cravings." *Complementary Therapies in Clinical Practice* 28 (2016): 136–145, doi:10.1016/j.ctcp.2017.06.004.

7. Stapleton, Peta and Doyle, Wava. "Mood and food cravings in overweight and obese Australian adults: Clues to treatment in food diaries." *Current Research in Psychology* 4, no.1 (2013): 6–15.

8. Stapleton., Peta et al. "Online group delivery of emotional freedom techniques for food cravings and weight management." *Cyberpsychology*, under review 2018.

9. Stapleton, Peta and Stewart, Michele. "Clinical EFT for food cravings in overweight adults: A comparison of in-person and online delivery of treatment." *Cogent Psychology*, under review, 2018.

10. Stapleton, Peta et al. "Emotional freedom techniques in the treatment of unhealthy eating behaviors and related psychological constructs in adolescents: A randomized controlled pilot trial." *Explore: The Journal of Science and Healing* 12, no. 2 (2016): 113–122.

11. Stapleton, Peta and Chatwin, Hannah. "How long does it take? 4-week versus 8-week emotional freedom, techniques

for food cravings in overweight adults." *OBM Integrative and Complementary Medicine* 3, no. 3 (2018): doi:10.21926/obm.icm.1803014.

Chapter 8

1. Martin, Andrew. *Building Classroom Success: Eliminating Academic Fear and Failure.* New York: Continuum International Publishing Group, 2010.

2. American Test Anxieties Association. Accessed November 1, 2017. http://amtaa.org.

3. Jones, S., Thornton, J., and Andrews, H. "Efficacy of EFT in reducing public speaking anxiety: A randomized controlled trial." *Energy Psychology: Theory, Research, and Treatment* 3, no. 1 (2011): 19–32.

4. Benor, Dan et al. "Pilot study of emotional freedom technique (eft), wholistic hybrid derived from EMDR and EFT (WHEE) and cognitive behavioral therapy (CBT) for treatment of test anxiety in university students." *Explore: The Journal of Science and Healing* 5, no. 6 (2009): 338–340.

5. Jain, S., and Rubino, A. "The effectiveness of emotional freedom techniques (EFT) for optimal test performance." *Energy Psychology: Theory, Research, and Treatment* 4 (2012): 13–24. doi:10.9769.EPJ.2012.4.2.SJ.

6. Rogers, R., and Sears, S. "Emotional freedom techniques (EFT) for stress in students: A randomized controlled dismantling study." *Energy Psychology: Theory, Research, and Treatment* 7, no. 2 (2015): 26–32. doi:10.9769/EPJ.2015.11.1.RR.

7. Boath, E., Stewart, A., and Carryer, A. "Is Emotional freedom techniques (EFT) generalizable? Comparing effects in sport science students versus complementary therapy students." *Energy Psychology: Theory, Research, and Treatment* 5, no. 2 (2013). doi:10.9769.EPJ.2013.5.2.EB.AC.AS.SU.

8. Boath, E., Stewart, A., and Carryer, A. "Tapping for success: A pilot study to explore if emotional freedom techniques (EFT) can reduce anxiety and enhance academic performance in university students." *Innovative Practice in Higher Education* 1, no. 3 (2013): 1–13.

9. Sezgin, N., and Ozcan, B. "The effect of progressive muscular relaxation and emotional freedom techniques on test anxiety in high school students: A randomized controlled." *Energy Psychology: Theory, Research, and Treatment* 1, no. 1 (2009): 23–30.

10. Aremu, A. O., and Taiwo, A. K. "Reducing mathematics anxiety among students with pseudo-dyscalculia in Ibadan through numerical cognition and emotional freedom techniques: Moderating effect of mathematics efficacy." *African Journal for the Psychological Studies of Social Issues* 17, no. 1 (2014): 113–129.

11. Stapleton, Peta et al. "Effectiveness of a school-based emotional freedom techniques intervention for promoting student well-being." *Adolescent Psychiatry* 7, no. 2 (2017): 112–126 doi:10.2174/2210676607666171101165425.

12. Martin, Andrew. *Building Classroom Success: Eliminating Academic Fear and Failure.* New York: Continuum International Publishing Group, 2010.

13. Gaesser, Amy, and Karan, Orv. "A randomized controlled comparison of emotional freedom technique and cognitive-behavioral therapy to reduce adolescent anxiety: A pilot study." *Journal of Alternative and Complementary Medicine* 23, no. 2 (2017): 102–108.

14. McCallion, Fiona. "Emotional freedom techniques for dyslexia: A case study." *Energy Psychology: Theory, Research, and Treatment* 4, no. 2 (2012). doi:10.9769/EPJ.2012.4.2.FM.

15. Church, Dawson. "The Effect of EFT (emotional freedom techniques) on athletic performance: A randomized controlled blind trial." *The Open Sports Sciences Journal* 2 (2009): 94–99.

16. Llewellyn-Edwards, T., and Llewellyn-Edwards, M. "The effect of EFT (emotional freedom techniques) on soccer performance." *Fidelity: Journal for the National Council of Psychotherapy* 47 (Spring 2012): 14–19.

17. Church, D., and Downs, D. "Sports confidence and critical incident intensity after a brief application of emotional freedom techniques: A pilot study." *The Sport Journal* 15 (2012).

18. Stapleton, Peta. *EFT for Teens.* California: Hay House, 2017.

Chapter 9

1. Kalla, Mahima and Khalil, Hanan. "The effectiveness of emotional freedom techniques (EFT) for improving the physical, mental, and emotional health of people with chronic diseases and/or mental health conditions: A systemic review protocol." *JBI Database of Systemic Reviews and Implementation Reports,* 12, no. 2 (2014): 114–124.

2. Kalla, Mahima et al. "Emotional freedom techniques (EFT) as a practice for supporting chronic disease health-care: A practitioners' perspective." *Disability and Rehabilitation* 40, no. 14 (2018): 1654–1662. doi:10.1080/09638288.2017.1306125.

3. Wells, Steve et al. "Evaluation of a meridian-based intervention, emotional freedom techniques (EFT), for reducing specific phobias of small animals." *Journal of Clinical Psychology* 59 (2003): 943–966.

4. Baker, A. H., and Siegel, L. S. "Emotional freedom techniques (EFT) reduce intense fears: A partial replication and extension of Wells, Polglase, Andrews, Carrington, & Baker (2003)." *Energy Psychology: Theory, Research, and Treatment* 2 (2010): 13–30. doi:10.9769.EPJ.2010.2.2.AHB.

5. Lambrou, P., Pratt, G., and Chevalier, G. "Physiological and psychological effects of a mind/body therapy on claustrophobia." *Journal of Subtle Energies and Energy Medicine* 14 (2005): 239–251.

6. Salas, M., Brooks, A., and Rowe, J. "The immediate effect of a brief energy psychology intervention (emotional freedom techniques) on specific phobias: A pilot study." *Explore: The Journal of Science and Healing* 7 (2011): 155–161.

7. Puspitaningrum, I., and Wijayanti, D. Y. "Effectiveness of spiritual emotional freedom technique (SEFT) intervention in schizophrenia with depression anxiety stress." Presented at Java International Nursing Conference, Semarang, October 6–7, 2012. Accessed January 18, 2018 from Diponegro University Institutional Repository: http://eprints.undip.ac.id/40379.

8. Moritz, S. et al. "Knock and it will be opened to you? An examination of meridian-tapping in obsessive compulsive disorder (OCD)." *Journal of Behavior Therapy & Experimental Psychiatry* 42 (2011): 81–88.

9. Church, Dawson and Brooks, Audrey. "The effect of EFT (emotional freedom techniques) on psychological symptoms in addiction treatment: A pilot study." *Journal of Scientific Research and Reports* 2, no. 2 (2013): 315–323.

10. Stapleton, Peta, Porter, Brett, and Sheldon, Terri. "Quitting smoking: How to use Emotional Freedom Techniques." *The International Journal of Healing and Caring* 13, no. 1. (2013): 1–16.

11. Hodge, P. M., & Jurgens, C. Y. "Psychological and physiological symptoms of psoriasis after group EFT (emotional freedom techniques) treatment: A pilot study." *Energy Psychology: Theory, Research, and Treatment* 3, no. 2 (2011): 13–23.

12. Jung Hwan Lee, Sun Yong Chung and Jong Woo Kim. "A Comparison of Emotional Freedom Techniques-Insomnia (EFT-I) and Sleep Hygiene Education (SHE) for Insomnia in a Geriatric Population: A Randomized Controlled Trial." *Journal of Energy Psychology: Theory, Research, and Treatment* 7, no.1 (2015): 22–29.

13. Babamahmoodi Abdolreza et al. "Emotional freedom technique (EFT) effects on psychoimmunological factors of chemically pulmonary injured veterans." *Iranian Journal of Allergy, Asthma and Immunology* [S.l.] 14, no. 1 (2015): 37–47, ISSN 1735-5249. http://ijaai.tums.ac.ir/index.php/ijaai/article/view/414.

14. Brattberg, Gunilla. "Self-administered EFT (emotional freedom techniques) in individuals with fibromyalgia: A randomized trial." *Integrative Medicine: A Clinician's Journal* 7, no. 4 (Aug/Sep 2008): 30–35.

15. Connais, C. "The effectiveness of emotional freedom technique on the somatic symptoms of fibromyalgia." Doctoral dissertation 3372777. University of the Rockies, Denver, CO, 2009.

16. Baker, B., and Hoffman, C. "Emotional Freedom Techniques (EFT) to reduce the side effects associated with tamoxifen and aromatase inhibitor use in women with breast cancer: A service evaluation." *European Journal of Integrative Medicine* 7, no. 2 (2014): 136–142. doi: 10.1016/j.eujim.2014.10.004.

17. Hajloo, M. et al. "Investigation on Emotional Freedom Technique effectiveness in diabetic patients' blood sugar control."

Mediterranean Journal of Social Sciences 5, no. 27 (2014): 1280. doi:10.5901/mjss.2014.v5n27p1280.

18. Church, D., and Palmer-Hoffman, J. "TBI symptoms improve after PTSD remediation with emotional freedom techniques." *Traumatology* 20, no. 3 (2014): 172–181.

19. Ortner, N., Palmer-Hoffman, J., and Clond, M. A. "Effects of emotional freedom techniques (EFT) on the reduction of chronic pain in adults: A pilot study." *Energy Psychology: Theory, Research, and Treatment* 6, no. 2 (2014): 14–21. doi:10.9769.EPJ.2014.6.2.NO.

20. Stapleton, Peta et al. "The lived experience of chronic pain and the impact of brief emotional freedom techniques (EFT) group therapy on coping." *Energy Psychology: Theory, Research, and Treatment* 8, no. 2 (2016): 18–28.

21. Church, Dawson. "Measuring physiological markers of emotional trauma: A randomized controlled trial of mind-body therapies." Paper presented at 10th annual Association for Comprehensive Energy Psychology (ACEP) conference, May 2008.

22. Church, D., and Nelms, J. "Pain, range of motion, and psychological symptoms in a population with frozen shoulder: A randomized controlled dismantling study of Clinical EFT (emotional freedom techniques)." *Archives of Scientific Psychology* 4, no. 1 (2016): 38–48. doi:10.1037/arc0000028.

23. Look, Carol. Improve Your Eyesight with EFT. 2006. http://vitalitylivingcollege.info/wp-content/uploads/2013/06/Improve-Your-Eyesight-EFT.pdf.

Chapter 10

1. Irgens, A. et al. "Thought Field Therapy compared to cognitive behavioral therapy and wait-list for agoraphobia: A randomized, controlled study with a 12-month follow-up." *Frontiers in Psychology* 8 (2017): 1027. doi:10.3389/fpsyg.2017.01027.

2. Folkes, C. "Thought field therapy and trauma recovery." *International Journal of Emergency Mental Health* 4 (2002): 99–103.

3. Sakai, C., Connolly, S., and Oas, P. "Treatment of PTSD in Rwanda genocide survivors using Thought Field Therapy." *International Journal of Emergency Mental Health* 12, no. 1 (2010): 41-49.

4. Connolly S., and Sakai C. "Brief trauma symptom intervention with Rwandan genocide-survivors using Thought Field Therapy." *International Journal of Emergency Mental Health* 13, no. 3 (2011): 161–172.

5. Connolly, S. M. et al. "Utilizing community resources to treat PTSD: A randomized controlled trial using Thought Field Therapy." *The African Journal of Traumatic Stress* 3, no. 1 (2013): 82–90.

6. Robson, R. H. et al. "Effectiveness of Thought Field Therapy provided by newly instructed community workers to a traumatized population in Uganda: A randomized trial." *Current Research in Psychology* 7, no.1 (2016): 1–11. doi:10.3844/crpsp.2016.1.11.

7. Edwards, Jenny and Vanchu-Orosco, M. "A meta-analysis of randomized and nonrandomized trials of Thought Field Therapy (TFT) for the treatment of post-traumatic stress disorder (PTSD)." Paper accepted at the Annual Meeting of the Association for Comprehensive Energy Psychology, San Antonio, Texas, 2017.

8. Schoninger, B., and Hartung, J. "Changes on Self-Report Measures of Public Speaking Anxiety Following Treatment with Thought Field Therapy." *Energy Psychology: Theory, Practice, and Research* 2, no. 1 (May 2010): 13–26.

9. Irgens, A. et al. "Thought Field Therapy (TFT) as a treatment for anxiety symptoms: A randomized controlled trial." *Explore: The Journal of Science and Healing* 8, no. 6 (2012): 331–337.

10. Irgens, A. et al. "Thought field therapy compared to cognitive behavioral therapy and wait-list for agoraphobia: A randomized, controlled study with a 12-month follow-up." *Frontiers in Psychology* 8 (2017): 1027. doi:10.3389/fpsyg.2017.01027.

11. Darby, D. W. "The efficacy of Thought Field Therapy as a treatment modality for individuals diagnosed with blood-injection-injury phobia." Dissertation Abstracts International, 64 (03), 1485B. (UMI No. 3085152), 2002.

12. Carbonell, J. "An experimental study of TFT and acrophobia." *The Thought Field* 2, no. 3 (1997): 1–6.

13. Pasahow, Robert. "Energy psychology and Thought Field Therapy in the treatment of tinnitus." *International Tinnitus Journal* 15, no. 2 (2009): 130–133.

14. Sakai, C. et al. "Thought Field Therapy clinical applications: Utilization in an HMO in behavioral medicine and behavioral health services." *Journal of Clinical Psychology* 57, no. 10 (2001): 1215–1227.

15. Yancey, V. "The use of Thought Field Therapy in educational settings." Dissertation Abstracts International 63 (07), 2470A. (UMI No. 3059661), 2002.

16. Callahan, Roger. "Raising and lowering HRV: Some clinical findings of Thought Field Therapy." *Journal of Clinical Psychology* 57, no. 10 (2001a): 1175–86.

17. Callahan, Roger. "The impact of Thought Field Therapy on heart rate variability." *Journal of Clinical Psychology* 57, no. 10 (2001b): 1153–1170.

18. Pignotti, M., and Steinberg, M. "Heart rate variability as an outcome measure for Thought Field Therapy in clinical practice." *Journal of Clinical Psychology* 57, no. 10 (2001): 1193–1206.

19. Herbert, J. D. and Gaudiano, B. A. "The search for the holy grail: Heart rate variability and Thought Field Therapy." *Journal of Clinical Psychology* 57, no. 10 (2001): 1207–1214. doi:10.1002/jclp.1087.

20. Metcalfe, Joannah. "Clinical case study: Thought Field Therapy." Base Formula: Well-being Inspired by Nature. November 11, 2017. https://www.baseformula.com/blog/clinical-case-study-thought-field-therapy.

21. Stewart, Anthony et al. "Can Matrix Reimprinting be effective in the treatment of emotional conditions in a public health setting? Results of a U.K. pilot study." *Energy Psychology: Theory, Research, and Treatment* 5, no.1 (2013): 13–31.

22. Boath, Elizabeth, Stewart, Anthony and Rolling, Caroline. "The impact of EFT and matrix reimprinting on the civilian survivors of war in Bosnia: A pilot study." *Current Research in Psychology* 5, no. 1 (2013): 64–72.

23. Crowther, Carol. "Sarah's Case Study Using EFT." Carol Crowther: Complementary Holistic Therapist and Trainer. http://www.eft-reiki.moonfruit.com/case-studies/4568075789.

24. Fitch, J., DiGirolamo, J. A., and Schmuldt, L. M. "The efficacy of primordial energy activation and transcendence (PEAT) for public speaking anxiety." *Energy Psychology: Theory, Research, and Treatment* 3, no. 2 (2011). doi:10.9769/EPJ.2011.3.2.JF.

25. Elder, C. et al. "Randomized trial of two mind–body interventions for weight-loss maintenance." *The Journal of Alternative and Complementary Medicine* 13, no. 1 (2007): 67–78. doi:10.1089/acm.2006.6237.

26. Elder C. et al. "Randomized trial of Tapas Acupressure Technique for weight loss maintenance." *BMC Complementary and Alternative Medicine* 15 (2012): 12–19. doi:10.1186/1472-6882-12-19.

Chapter 11

1. Mind Heart Connect. "The Tapping Journal." http://www.mindheartconnect.com/product/the-tapping-journal.

2. Lis, Valerie. "10 Common Mistakes in Tapping: Resolving Them Leads to Exceptional Results." *EFT Universe.* Accessed January 30, 2018. http://www.eftuniverse.com/refinements-to-eft/10-common-mistakes-in-tapping-resolving-them-leads-to-exceptional-results.

INDEX

emotional learnings and, 44
learning disabilities and, 162
memory consolidation theory for,
34, 44–47, 67–68, 80–81, 91, 158
Movie Technique for, 18–20, 23, 228
phobias and fears and, 182–183
smoking and, 186–187
table analogy for, 16–17
triggers for, 14–15, 22–23

Pavlov, Ivan, 67

phobias and fears. *See also* anxiety and
anxiety EFT research; *specific fears
and phobias*
about, xxvii–xxviii, 174
aspects of, 14
behavioral kinesiology for, 27
childhood trauma and, 181–183
comparison studies, 43, 147–149,
155–156
dismantling studies, 49–50
memory reconsolidation theory on,
67–68
physiological changes and, 38, 43
research on, 174–179
sexual abuse and, 71–74
in students, 146–153. *See also* failure, fear of
Thought Field Therapy for, 214–218,
220
trauma (general) and, 180–181
treatment length for, 42

physical abuse, 58, 66, 91–92

physiological changes, from tapping.
See also brain imaging
about, xix, 12–13
in central nervous system, 39–41
cognitive shifts, 7
eyesight issues, 207–208
heart rate variability studies, 39–41,
166–167, 177, 221–222
mirror neurons and, 18
misconceptions of, 240
with phobias, 38, 43
with PTSD, xxvi
somatic interventions and, 33–34
stress hormones and, xxviii, 33–34,
36, 39, 41, 78. *See also* cortisol

placebo effect, defined, 48

positive affirmations, 7, 9, 235–236,
242–243

post-traumatic stress disorder. *See* PTSD
and PTSD EFT research

Primordial Energy Activation and Transcendence (PEAT), 229–230

prisoner studies, 66

procrastination, 16

progressive muscle relaxation (PMR),
184–185

psoriasis, 190–191

psychotherapy
comparison studies, 32–35
effectiveness of, 32
history of, xxiii–xxv

PTSD and PTSD EFT research, 57–74.
See also trauma (general)
about, xxvi, 58–59
athletes and, 166–167
brain imaging and, 35
CNS effects of, 40–41
comparison studies, 59–64, 211–212
delivery method research, 61–62
EFT as mechanism of change for,
66–68
EFT clinical guidelines, 68–71
gene expression studies, 39
intervention reviews, 64–65
meta-analysis on, 213
other tapping techniques for, xxviii,
209–213, 220, 226–229
phobias and, 180–181
sexual abuse and, 57–58, 71–74
somatic therapy for, 35–37
traumatic brain injuries and,
197–198
treatment length, 42, 68
veterans and, 39, 59–64, 66, 67, 74

PTSD Checklist (PCL), 61, 68–71, 212,
226–227

public-speaking anxiety, xxviii, 86–87,
147, 150–153, 213–214, 229–230

pulmonary issues, 192–193

p-value, defined, 52–53

R

Ramachandran, V. S., 18

randomized studies, defined, 48

ACKNOWLEDGMENTS

....

This journey started in May 2017 when I was having coffee with a colleague, and he said, "You should write a book." I laughed and asked, "What am I going to write a book on?" He replied something about the science and research behind tapping. I laughed again and said, "I don't have time to write a book."

Apparently I did, and this is it. And it truly would not have been possible without the support of many people behind and in front of the scene. In no particular order (except maybe the first one), I want to send my heartfelt thanks to all of the following people:

To my husband, Wayde, for entertaining the girls when I had to barricade the office on weekends when writing. Lucky for me he can cook too.

To my daughters, Megan and Elise. They keep me light and laughing with all this science, and didn't mind me asking questions like, "How do you tell your friends about tapping?"

To the whole Hay House team, especially Reid Tracy and Leon Nacson, Patty Gift, Nicolette Young, and Sally Mason-Swaab. They put full trust in me to deliver this book, and I am truly grateful for the opportunity. A very special, heartfelt thank-you to Louise Hay, who started it all. What many people won't know (unless they read this) is that the day I signed the Hay House publishing contract was the same day Louise died. While I didn't ever think I would meet her, I had a quiet moment when I heard the news and asked for her blessing to join her publishing family. Within the hour I was getting out of my car and looked down to see an enormous white feather on my shoe. Rationally, I don't know where this would have come from as I was driving, but perhaps it was a nod from Louise.

To several Hay House authors who have become friends and constantly offered their support: Dr. David Hamilton, Nick Ortner, and Dr. Joe Dispenza (especially for the Foreword!).

To the many people in my life who have been the cheerleaders and never once doubted I could do this (even when I was going around in circles)—my sisters, Kate and Anna, and brother, Andrew; my rock-solid partner in Mind Heart Connect, Kate; the fabulous Dr. Lori Leyden; Sandy Coventry, for her magic on the images and figures; and my parents, who keep asking, "How's the book?" In addition, there have been so many practitioners and therapists, EFT leaders and pioneers who have always been a source of support and inspiration, and to all of them, I say thank you.

To the giants in the EFT world who always answer my e-mails and questions (and sometimes there are many!): Dr. Dawson Church and John Freedom—thank you!

To a few very special people who read the manuscript and offered their expert opinions and thoughts: Dr. David Feinstein and Dr. Craig Weiner. When writing, it is often difficult to see the whole forest of trees, and I am truly grateful for their wisdom.

To the practitioners and clients who offered their stories—without these the picture of how and why EFT works is incomplete. They are the ones who allow us to conduct trials and ask them the same questions over and over to determine any changes!

To all the researchers who have been pioneers in conducting trials and publishing their outcomes in an area that is unconventional and fourth wave! We need leaders who will do this in order to move a field forward, and I am humbled by what I have learned along the way.

And finally, to Alan, who is no longer with us but was the person who said I should learn this weird tapping thing and showed me this path; and to J.D., who set the wheels in motion for this book to come to life. Thank you.

ABOUT THE AUTHOR

Dr. Peta Stapleton is a registered clinical and health psychologist and associate professor at Bond University (Queensland, Australia). Peta specializes in eating disorders and emotional eating, women's health, and adolescent issues, and she is a world leader and researcher in Emotional Freedom Techniques. She has been awarded the Harvey Baker Research Award for meticulous research in energy psychology by the Association of Comprehensive Energy Psychology (ACEP), and also the greatest contribution to the field of Energy Psychology by ACEP.

Peta is a director of Mind Heart Connect™, an organization to raise awareness of the mind-body-heart connect through evidence-based practices. She is also the creator of Tapping in the Classroom®, a research-inspired online training for teachers worldwide to learn EFT for daily classroom use.

Peta is a publication machine and likes to conduct world-first trials, even though she is an introvert at heart. No one really believes this, though. Peta is married with two daughters and calls Queensland home. It's a lot like California with the sunny skies, but way less traffic.

We hope you enjoyed this Hay House book. If you'd like to receive our online catalog featuring additional information on Hay House books and products, or if you'd like to find out more about the Hay Foundation, please contact:

Hay House, Inc., P.O. Box 5100, Carlsbad, CA 92018-5100
(760) 431-7695 or (800) 654-5126
(760) 431-6948 (fax) or (800) 650-5115 (fax)
www.hayhouse.com® • www.hayfoundation.org

———

Published in Australia by: Hay House Australia Pty. Ltd.,
18/36 Ralph St., Alexandria NSW 2015
Phone: 612-9669-4299 • *Fax:* 612-9669-4144
www.hayhouse.com.au

Published in the United Kingdom by: Hay House UK, Ltd.,
The Sixth Floor, Watson House, 54 Baker Street, London W1U 7BU
Phone: +44 (0)20 3927 7290 • *Fax:* +44 (0)20 3927 7291
www.hayhouse.co.uk

Published in India by: Hay House Publishers India,
Muskaan Complex, Plot No. 3, B-2, Vasant Kunj, New Delhi 110 070
Phone: 91-11-4176-1620 • *Fax:* 91-11-4176-1630
www.hayhouse.co.in

———

<u>Access New Knowledge.</u>
<u>Anytime. Anywhere.</u>

Learn and evolve at your own pace
with the world's leading experts.

www.hayhouseU.com

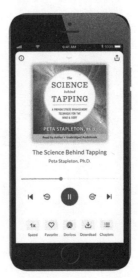